Culture of Health in Practice

Culture of Health in Practice

Innovations in Research, Community Engagement, and Action

ALONZO L. PLOUGH

OXFORD
UNIVERSITY PRESS

OXFORD
UNIVERSITY PRESS

Oxford University Press is a department of the University of Oxford. It furthers
the University's objective of excellence in research, scholarship, and education
by publishing worldwide. Oxford is a registered trade mark of Oxford University
Press in the UK and certain other countries.

Published in the United States of America by Oxford University Press
198 Madison Avenue, New York, NY 10016, United States of America.

Library of Congress Cataloging-in-Publication Data
Names: Sharing Knowledge to Build a Culture of Health Conference
(2018 : Chandler, Ariz.), author. | Plough, Alonzo L., editor.
Title: Culture of health in practice : innovations in research, community
engagement, and action / [edited by] Alonzo L. Plough.
Other titles: Robert Wood Johnson Foundation culture of health series ; 3.
Identifiers: LCCN 2019044747 (print) | LCCN 2019044748 (ebook) |
ISBN 9780190071400 (hb) | ISBN 9780190071424 (epub) |
ISBN 9780190071431 (online)
Subjects: MESH: Health Equity | Social Determinants of Health |
Cultural Diversity | United States | Congress
Classification: LCC RA418 (print) | LCC RA418 (ebook) |
NLM W 76 AA1 | DDC 362.1–dc23
LC record available at https://lccn.loc.gov/2019044747
LC ebook record available at https://lccn.loc.gov/2019044748

This material is not intended to be, and should not be considered, a substitute for medical or other
professional advice. Treatment for the conditions described in this material is highly dependent on the
individual circumstances. And, while this material is designed to offer accurate information with respect
to the subject matter covered and to be current as of the time it was written, research and knowledge about
medical and health issues is constantly evolving and dose schedules for medications are being revised
continually, with new side effects recognized and accounted for regularly. Readers must therefore always
check the product information and clinical procedures with the most up-to-date published product
information and data sheets provided by the manufacturers and the most recent codes of conduct and safety
regulation. The publisher and the authors make no representations or warranties to readers, express or
implied, as to the accuracy or completeness of this material. Without limiting the foregoing, the publisher
and the authors make no representations or warranties as to the accuracy or efficacy of the drug dosages
mentioned in the material. The authors and the publisher do not accept, and expressly disclaim,
any responsibility for any liability, loss, or risk that may be claimed or incurred as a consequence of the
use and/or application of any of the contents of this material.

1 3 5 7 9 8 6 4 2
Printed by LSC Communications, United States of America

CONTENTS

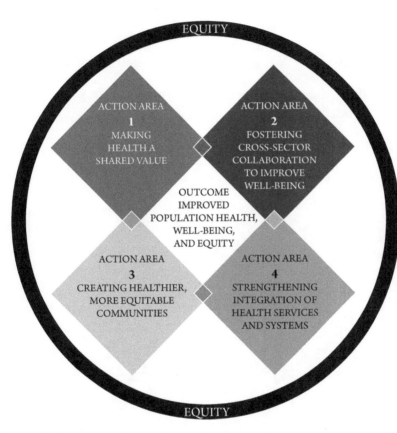

Figure 0.1 Culture of Health Action Framework

Introduction

When a tribal elder offered a traditional Native American blessing to open the Robert Wood Johnson Foundation's third annual *Sharing Knowledge to Build a Culture of Health* conference on the Gila River Indian Community in Arizona, audience members recognized that the choice of location was an essential component of the conference. They would be part of an event that would be framed around equity and extend well beyond the usual boundaries of an academic conference. In February 2018, on lands that indigenous peoples have long held sacred, in a state with a complex cultural history and a strong sense of place, researchers, policymakers, practitioners, and advocates gathered to talk about advancing a Culture of Health.

Participants brought a variety of training experiences, background knowledge, and personal experiences with them, along with the unique perspectives they had gained by working across academic, government, clinical, and community settings, in rural and urban milieus, as well as with the many and varied populations who live in the United States. This intersectionality—on display both at the *Sharing Knowledge* conference and in this book—underscores the importance of achieving health equity throughout this country, which is the crosscutting focus of how the Robert Wood Johnson Foundation (RWJF) is advancing a Culture of Health.

> *Health equity means that everyone has a fair and just opportunity to be healthier. This requires removing obstacles to health such as poverty, discrimination, and their consequences, including powerlessness and lack of access to good jobs with fair pay, quality education and housing, safe environments, and health care.*—Robert Wood Johnson Foundation definition[1]

The abundant data that document health inequities in housing, education, incarceration, income, opportunity, and so much else in the United States are a challenge for our work and the nation as a whole. Although it is essential to continue

Culture of Health in Practice, Alonzo L. Plough. Oxford University Press (2020) © Robert Wood Johnson Foundation
DOI: 10.1093/oso/9780190071400.001.0001

refining our understanding of the scale of the problem, the Foundation is increasingly dedicated to figuring out how to solve it. Addressing the historical and enduring structures of racism is central to that effort. Given all that we know about which groups inequity harms most, many of the conference presenters explicitly acknowledged and confronted the imperative of tackling racism head on.

The 2018 *Sharing Knowledge* conference came at a challenging moment in American history, when reductions in health care coverage, the loss of funding to tackle social determinants of health, and the growing risks associated with climate change have all hit vulnerable populations first and hardest. Meanwhile, life expectancy for the nation has been on a sustained decline for the first time since the early 20th century, when it was accompanied by the twin disasters of the flu pandemic and World War I.[2]

Polarization, evident in our civic discourse, has intensified these challenges. An underlying tenet of a Culture of Health is that "we are all in this together," yet a great deal of suspicion is separating disparate groups of people. Until we can find a place of trust, it will be difficult to have the reasoned discussions and reach the shared understandings that can drive progress toward common goals.

Fortunately, there are countervailing forces that open up space for optimism. The contributors to this volume have much to tell us about the value of rigorous scholarship, innovative practice, and inclusive community action to promote health and well-being for all. These change-makers are testing, implementing, and evaluating transformative solutions to long-standing problems, especially at regional and local levels. With their focus on root causes and collaboration, they are reminding us that in any sociopolitical environment opportunities exist to scale and spread ideas that can help advance health equity. Among the themes that emerge clearly here is that hope, determination, and evidence have power.

The imperative of connecting across our differences surfaced again and again at the conference. One of the great strengths of our time together was the opportunity for both structured and spontaneous exchanges, which took place on the podium, during the question-and-answer period that accompanied every session, and informally at meals and receptions. People who have lived experiences with the issues being explored, individuals who are studying those issues, and others who are part of the systems and institutions that can be redesigned to address them shared their ideas frankly but respectfully. This book tries to capture some of the excitement in those provocative and useful interactions.

At RWJF, we increasingly recognize the role that narrative can play in promoting a Culture of Health. The stories a society tells often become the basis of the policies it crafts. How we depict people who become addicted to opioids or reside in isolated rural pockets influences what we do to and for them. Anecdotes about families who apply for public benefits, or individuals who emerge from prisons, help determine whether societal resources will be used to support or punish them. The contributors to this volume offer both data and personal insight to help us consider the structural constraints and conditions that often shape individual behavior and the strategies that can lift up populations.

No single chapter here is dedicated specifically to health equity, just as that subject was not the exclusive provenance of any one conference session, because we recognize its centrality in all that we examine. The pursuit of health equity propels RWJF forward and informs every section of this book, which is organized as follows:

Section I, "Embracing the Cultural Dimension in a Culture of Health," lifts up the strengths that sustain well-being in so many cultures in the United States, despite their historical and contemporary marginalization. America is a land of extraordinary diversity, but we rarely focus on the assets intrinsic to cultural identity and the contribution to the nation's well-being that this diversity brings. Media is one of the tools through which this story can be told, and plays a vital role in advancing a productive narrative. Celebrating the contributions of the nation's many cultures and recognizing the wide reach of media give us new ways to think about connectivity as a driving force for health and well-being.

Section II, "At Home, at School, at Work," calls attention to the places where people spend much of their time and shows how each setting has the power to promote health, or to undermine it. Social cohesion and a sense of belonging are important constituents of any healthy community, but in some regions, decades of disinvestment have shattered those bonds. Strengthening the institutions that can help revitalize towns and neighborhoods, grow stable families, and educate youth, as well as recognizing employers who act in the interest of their workers are affirmative measures that can help repair those bonds.

Section III, "Complex Challenges, Inventive Solutions," takes on a broad range of interconnected topics that have drawn considerable attention from many fields and brought new perspectives to the table. Mass incarceration, climate change, addiction, and immigration are societal issues with long histories—they did not surface suddenly, nor will they quickly be resolved—but some have become particular flashpoints in this time of acrimony. Deconstructing myths, engaging in evidence-guided dialogue, telling stories, and lifting up our common humanity all advance health-promoting strategies and help span social and ideological divides.

As the conference in Arizona drew to a close, participants left with stacks of business cards from new colleagues and potential collaborators. Their conference evaluations tell us they were bursting with ideas and had a deeper understanding of the dynamic interplay across sectors that is so essential to a Culture of Health. This book continues the conversation that began in the arid desert clime of Phoenix, when a group that included educators and hospital administrators, scholars and military officers, criminal justice professionals and health care providers, community organizers, and environmental advocates—to name just a handful of the participants—joined to talk about the meaning of health and well-being, and how best to foster them.

MAINSTREAMING A CULTURE OF HEALTH

How a Culture of Health Can Become Normative

> *In a Culture of Health, all people in American understand that we're in this together—no one is excluded. Everyone has access to the care they need and a fair and just opportunity to make healthier choices. In a Culture of Health, communities flourish and individuals thrive.—Robert Wood Johnson Foundation*

"No culture can live if it attempts to be exclusive." The ideas behind those words are as important today as they were when Mahatma Gandhi spoke them in 1959.[1] A Culture of Health requires respecting the many cultural traditions that enrich America and a discourse that honors our differences as it advances our common interests. Thoughtful dialogue will help us fulfill the promise of providing fair and just opportunity to all.

The chapters in the opening section of this book help us consider how to do that. Celebrating cultural diversity and shifting the public conversation are two cornerstones of a Culture of Health. Neither is tied to a single policy or discipline, making each useful in helping people of all backgrounds, viewpoints, and regions think across our silos and beyond our blinders. They acknowledge areas of deep division, but they also suggest opportunities for repairing damage and healing wounds.

"Incorporating 'Culture' Within a Culture of Health" draws on the values of two vibrant populations that are especially prominent in the conference setting of Arizona—Hispanics and Native Americans. Each has much to contribute to the health and well-being of all groups of people, and their experiences suggest areas of study and practice that can help share and scale their contributions.

The chapter opens with population health data indicating that Hispanics live longer and have certain health advantages when it comes to chronic health conditions, and it explores possible sources of those advantages. The chapter continues with a portrait of one agency that seamlessly grounds behavioral health, employment, and housing services in deeply held Native traditions. Drumming ceremonies, sweat lodges, and other Native customs are among the strategies used to deliver evidence-based services that promote well-being and redress a history of policies aimed at undermining Native people and values.

"How Media Shapes the Public Discourse and Influences Health" describes the multiple roles of modern media in determining not only what consumers know, but also how and what they think. The exponential growth of ideologically driven cable channels and social media, dovetailing with cutbacks in newspaper staffing and coverage, point to the many ways that the power and reach of media are shifting even as they continue to reshape American society and norms.

In this environment, multiple media compete for viewers, readers, and listeners who will click on their websites, buy their products, sign their petitions, and often accept their spin, especially if it reinforces personal perspectives. Thoughtful information about complex public health issues is easily lost in that context, leading too many people to base their decision-making on incomplete, biased, and even inaccurate information.

At a time when so many Americans feel disenfranchised or ignored, the chapters of *Mainstreaming a Culture of Health* show us that we are indeed "all in this together." When we appreciate our cultural diversity, we are better able to understand who we are, connect with one another, and move forward together. If we can find ways to tell and share our stories honestly and with respect, we will move farther down the path toward a Culture of Health.

Incorporating "Culture" Within a Culture of Health

John M. Ruiz, PhD, Associate Professor, Director of Social Risk & Resilience Factors (SuRRF) Lab, Director of the Health Psychology Track, University of Arizona

Diana Yazzie Devine, MBA, President and Chief Executive Officer, Native American Connections

The pathway to greater equity and better health outcomes for individuals in America of all cultures starts with the recognition that people from every background have contributions to make. When people feel connected to their own cultural values and respect the unique perspectives of their neighbors, co-workers, and acquaintances, regardless of their origins and ancestry, individuals and communities are more likely to thrive.

> *As a source of exchange, innovation, and creativity, cultural diversity is as necessary for humankind as biodiversity is for nature.* —UNESCO *Universal Declaration on Cultural Diversity*

Yet culture has tended to be underemphasized as a potent force in a Culture of Health. "We can learn so much by exploring different cultural approaches to supporting health and well-being," said Karabi B. Acharya, ScD, MHS, director of RWJF's Global Ideas for U.S. Solutions team. "We need to dig in more deeply on 'culture' in our effort to build a Culture of Health."

The increasing diversity of America underscores the need to change that. Thirty-nine percent of the nation's population is now nonwhite, and demographers predict the United States will be a majority-minority country

Culture of Health in Practice, Alonzo L. Plough. Oxford University Press (2020) © Robert Wood Johnson Foundation
DOI: 10.1093/oso/9780190071400.001.0001

by 2045.[1] Inclusivity is essential if we are to broaden the conversation and strengthen the institutions that surround and shape our lives. But the data tell us we are far from doing all that is possible to gather America's many cultures at the same table.

For example, a disproportionate share of research endeavors and policy decisions come from only one culture: whites of European descent. According to the National Center for Education Statistics, more than 75 percent of full-time faculty in degree-granting postsecondary institutions in 2016 were white, and 10 percent were Asian/Pacific Islanders. Blacks and Hispanics each made up just 5 percent of the total.[2]

The halls of government show much the same thing. Although cultural diversity in the U.S. House of Representatives and Senate has increased significantly in recent years, only 22 percent of Congress members are racial or ethnic minorities.[3] Still, the 116th Congress is the most diverse in history, suggesting that at least some elements of the power structure may be beginning to shift.

The setting of this *Sharing Knowledge* conference offered a unique opportunity for participants to spend time thinking about the "culture" side of a Culture of Health. The modern hotel where the convening took place is sited on lands owned by the Gila River Indian community, home to the Akimel O'odham (Pima) people as far back as 300 B.C., and to the Piipaash (Maricopa) people who joined them in the mid-1700s.

The surrounding state has grown rapidly over the past few decades, with the population increasing by more than 12 percent between 2010 and 2018 alone. About 55 percent of Arizona's 7.1 million people are white, and nearly one-third are Hispanic. Native peoples and blacks each make up about 5 percent of the population, and Asians 3.5 percent. More than one-quarter (27%) of Arizonans speak a language other than English at home.[4]

This chapter takes that rich mix as its starting point and zooms in to consider how the deeply held values of Hispanic and Native peoples promote equity and a Culture of Health within Arizona and beyond. John Ruiz describes the "Hispanic paradox"—an unexpected relationship between health risks and mortality rates—and suggests that Hispanic values of collectivism and social integration can inform health policy and practice. Diana Yazzie Devine demonstrates how Native traditions and values ground evidence-based practices in behavioral health, substance use, housing, and other services.

As we dive into that conversation, it is important to bring to the forefront the complex and often delicate issue of the words we use to talk about different cultures; see "A Note About Language" at the end of this chapter for a perspective on this central issue.

The "Hispanic Paradox"

As a graduate student in psychology, John Ruiz's first and formative research experience was interviewing traumatized residents of Oklahoma City within 24 hours of the 1995 bombing. That experience convinced him that psychological factors are associated with physiological characteristics in ways that have implications for health.

Ruiz recalled that this interest in Hispanic health was piqued when he discovered that literature on the issue "was just blank." One analysis of top articles published in behavioral science journals between 2003 and 2007 found that 96 percent of research participants were from the United States or other Western industrialized countries. Although those countries constitute only 15 percent of the world's population, many health conclusions are drawn from this limited and unrepresentative sample.[5]

The failure to include Hispanics in research is especially disturbing given that they are the largest nonwhite ethnic group in the United States, with an estimated population of almost 59 million (18.1% of the population).[6] Nearly two-thirds (65%) were born in the United States, and 11 percent are naturalized citizens.[7]

Their families hail from many places. Almost two-thirds (63.4%) have Mexican roots, with the remainder from Puerto Rico (9.5%), Central America (9.2%), South America (6.0%), and Cuba (3.7%).[8] Although they may share a common language and some of the same values, their traditions, norms, and even diets vary considerably.

Social Supports Eclipse Health Risks

The Hispanic mortality paradox is the epidemiological phenomenon where Hispanics experience lower mortality and better health relative to non-Hispanic whites despite disproportionately greater socioeconomic risk. —
John M. Ruiz

Data from the Office of Minority Health at the U.S. Department of Health and Human Services indicate that Hispanics are at greater health risk than whites. Among psychosocial risk factors, they have less education than whites (66% of Hispanics living in the United States vs. 92% of whites have a high school diploma). In 2015, 19.5 percent of Hispanics lacked health insurance (ranging from a high of 28.2% of Central Americans to a low of 8.5% of Puerto Ricans), compared with 6.3 percent of whites. The Hispanic poverty rate, at 22.6 percent, is more than twice that of whites (10.4%), and median household income was $44,782 compared with $61,394 for whites.[9]

Physical health risks are significant as well. Data from the Centers for Disease Control and Prevention (CDC) indicate that 78.5 percent of Hispanics are overweight or obese (compared with 68.5% of whites). Just over 12 percent have diagnosed diabetes (vs. 6.7% of whites).[10] They also have high rates of undiagnosed or poorly managed diseases and give their own health and the quality of their health care low ratings.

And yet, persuasive data demonstrate that, by and large, Hispanics live longer and have fewer hospital and emergency department visits, as well as a lower incidence of some diseases, even after controlling for age, gender, and country of origin. Although the statistics differ somewhat among Hispanics by place of origin, Ruiz characterizes those distinctions as "shades of good," with advantages among all subgroups, compared with non-Hispanic whites.

Among the highlights:

- **Hispanics in America live three years longer than whites, and almost seven years longer than blacks.** Life expectancy for Hispanics born in 2015 is 81.9 years, compared with 78.7 years for whites and 75.5 years for blacks born that year.[11]
- **Hispanics have a lower incidence of common forms of cancer and cardiovascular disease and are less likely to die from these conditions.** Their rates of prostrate, breast, and lung cancer are lower than those of whites. Hispanics smoke significantly less than whites and blacks. Prevalence rates for stroke and hypertension are similar to those for whites but significantly lower than those for blacks. Hispanics do have more diabetes than whites.[12]
- **Hispanic infant mortality rates are similar to those of whites.** Despite socioeconomic disparities and differences in access to and quality of prenatal care, infant mortality among Hispanics in 2016 was 5 deaths per 1,000 live births, compared with 4.9 deaths per 1,000 live births for whites.[13] Infant mortality rates among Hispanics vary by place of origin, however, ranging from 3 deaths per 1,000 live births among Cubans to 7.2 deaths per 1,000 live births among Puerto Ricans.[14] Hispanics overall are less likely to have low birthweight babies than whites, although the rate among Puerto Ricans is twice that of whites.[15]
- **The edge in longevity and some health advantages is more pronounced for foreign-born and less acculturated Hispanics, those living in dense Hispanic neighborhoods, and older people.** Studies of Hispanics conclude that those with greater connection to their language, food, customs, and values live longer and have certain health advantages, such as lower risks of some common diseases and greater survival rates in the context of disease, than those who were born here, emigrated at a younger age, and are more acculturated.[16]

The longer Hispanics live in the U.S. and the more they acculturate to U.S. culture, the less pronounced are the differences in longevity. —John M. Ruiz

Overcoming Doubts About the Findings

As the paradox garnered attention in the health field, it attracted a lot of controversy. Hypotheses surfaced to suggest that only healthier Hispanics come to America (the "healthy migrant" hypothesis) or that Hispanics return to their countries of origin as they age (the "salmon bias" hypothesis). These were set aside, however, after further analysis, Ruiz said. Moreover, the health paradox is not limited to Hispanics. Chapter 8, "Achieving Health Equity for Immigrants and Their Children," notes a broader "immigrant paradox," in which immigrants from other parts of the world also realize some health advantages compared with native-born Americans and native-born members of their own ethnic group.

Questions arose about the methodology underlying the findings of the Hispanic paradox and about possible characteristics of Hispanics that could explain the findings. "Science likes good questions," said Ruiz, as he set out to look for answers. He explored two alternative explanations, one methodological, the other focused on the use of health care services.

A Second Look at the Methodology

Many in the field questioned the accuracy of the estimation methodology used to identify the paradox, which relies on death certificates and census data to ascertain life expectancy for each racial and ethnic group. Indeed, for many years the CDC put an asterisk next to its figures about Hispanic longevity, noting possible problems with the data. Using the estimation methodology, researchers found that Hispanics had a 20 percent chance of living longer than whites.

To explore this concern, researchers looked for flaws in the estimation methodology. In one study published in 2011, they compared death certificates with survey information taken from the Current Population Survey for the years 1979 to 1998. They found that the mortality paradox could not be explained by differences in the classification of Hispanics used on death certificates and the survey results.[17]

Ruiz tested the paradox by employing a methodology that didn't rely on estimation data. Through a meta-analysis, he examined patient outcomes from 58 studies involving 4.6 million people who were tracked longitudinally. "This gets around the problem with estimation data in that you are following specific individuals over time," he explained.

Using this approach, Ruiz found that Hispanics were 17.5 percent more likely to be alive at the end of the studies, compared with non-Hispanics.[18] "Two very different methodologies got us to essentially the same ballpark," he added, noting that as of 2018, CDC longevity data no longer include the qualifying asterisk.

A Look at Health Care Utilization

Next, Ruiz and his team sought to examine whether these ethnic advantages were limited to mortality or whether they extended to overall physical health. Ruiz verified that the life span differential for Arizona's Hispanic population mirrored the national differential every year from 2008 to 2015. Then the team examined hospital utilization trends—which are good barometers of the health of a population—among Hispanics and whites. The goal was to examine whether the Hispanic paradox was evident in hospital use within the context of the verified mortality advantage.

Based on inpatient admissions, emergency department visits, and discharge data from Arizona hospitals for 2008 to 2015, coupled with results from the American Community Survey[19] for those years, Ruiz found:

- **Hispanics were less likely than whites to be admitted to hospitals for every year studied.** In 2015, for example, Hispanics had fewer than 60 inpatient admissions per 1,000 Hispanic people, compared with about 130 admissions per 1,000 white people living in Arizona. The differential in admissions held for all ages (18 to 64) and for all payer sources: Medicare, Medicaid, private insurance, and no insurance.
- **Hispanics visited emergency departments less frequently than whites.** In 2015, Hispanics had about 225 emergency department visits per 1,000 Hispanic people, compared with almost 275 visits per 1,000 whites.

In a separate analysis, Ruiz found that Hispanics had lower rates of hospital inpatient and emergency room deaths than whites every year between 2011 and 2015.

> The health effects are broad, significant, robust, and replicated. —John M. Ruiz

Thus, the Arizona data offer additional support for lower population mortality, lower hospital admission, lower emergency department usage, and lower mortality in those hospital settings. The differences were quite large and held for all ages and insurance categories, said Ruiz. Although not definitive, he added, the data strongly support the hypothesis of a broader Hispanic health paradox.

With the controversies largely put to rest, Ruiz turned next to exploring reasons for the Hispanic health advantage.

Cultural Values: *Familismo, Simpatico, Respeto*

The Hispanic paradox "opened my eyes" to the possibility that people at even high health risk can achieve equal or better health outcomes than people with substantially lower risk, Ruiz said. "There must be some offsetting resilience that comes into play." To explore the source of such resilience, Ruiz drew from existing literature suggesting that social support leads to better health outcomes.

In Ruiz's view, Western medicine's health frame emphasizes risk and risk reduction. Although that has led to important medical advances, he argued that the Hispanic paradox suggests a paradigm that includes resilience factors may help to advance understanding of health and well-being.

A history of research on the connection between mortality and social relationships provides some support for that argument. One broad study of mortality found that "people with stronger social relationships had a 50 percent increased likelihood of survival than those with weaker social relationships."[20]

Researchers often express values that facilitate health-promoting social relationships as *familismo* (valuing family), *simpatica/o* (valuing social harmony), and *respeto* (respect and investment in caring for older people).[21]

These values endure over the course of a lifetime and contribute to a tight social fabric that may confer resilience even in the face of risk. In infancy, this social fabric manifests in large caregiver networks. In daily life, it provides communal coping resources—the problem is not "mine," it is "ours"—that diffuse feelings of stress. In times of illness, it delivers caregiving and encourages receptivity to accepting services, and in old age it confers respect and continued engagement in family activities.

If cultural norms such as these are key factors in Hispanic health advantages, Ruiz hypothesized, then the more Hispanics retain their cultures—the less acculturated they are—the healthier they should be. After examining studies of health outcomes of Hispanics living in dense ethnic neighborhoods or "barrios," that is exactly the pattern that emerges. As noted, health benefits are greater for Hispanics living in barrios, for foreign-born Hispanics, for those who were older when they immigrated here, and for those who are less acculturated to American life.

Ruiz found additional evidence in the "halo" effect—a phenomenon in which non-Hispanics living in or near Hispanic neighborhoods show health advantages similar to those of Hispanics. One study concluded, "The health benefits of living in Hispanic areas appear to bridge ethnic divides, resulting in better birth outcomes even for those of non-Hispanic origin."[22] This evidence suggests that at least some of the resilience is due to social factors from which non-Hispanics who are proximal to Hispanics can benefit.

Ruiz proposed two cornerstones of Hispanic collectivism as ripe for further research, policy, and practice: the experience of stress and the receptivity to offers of help.

Responses to Stress

Research has shown that although Hispanics, along with other low-income or marginalized populations, are *exposed* to more stressors in their lives compared with non-Hispanic whites, they may actually *experience* less stress. "Social baseline theory," for example, holds that the degree of closeness to others affects how people perceive the personal toll of a given situation.[23]

Ruiz noted that studies have reported that Hispanics show "a decreased physiological response to stress relative to other minority groups and non-Hispanic whites." He posits that collectivism buffers stress levels by altering how people appraise stress and by diffusing coping from the individual to the social network. One study concluded that "familialism [another way to express familismo] was positively correlated with support and negatively correlated with stress and pregnancy anxiety . . . and that the associations of familialism with social support and stress were significantly stronger among Latinas than European Americans."[24]

Responses to Offers of Help

Ruiz uses cell biology to explain how *familismo, simpatico,* and *respeto* might contribute to health outcomes. In order for an effect to be realized, he said, a signal (in this case, an offer of help) must be sent, and a receptor (here, openness to help) must accept the signal. Many Western health and social interventions focus on the first part and overlook the second. "Hispanics are very good at this second part," Ruiz believes. "They expect support to be offered and when it comes, they take it. Together, this provision and acceptance creates an effect."

Questions Remain

The body of research that documents the mortality paradox—Hispanics do indeed live longer and healthier lives—also suggests the causes are cultural, not clinical. The closer they remain to their values and traditions, the more likely they are to enjoy better health.

But a deeper understanding is essential, especially since the contradiction between the high health risks and significant health advantages of Hispanics complicates accepted wisdom. Indeed, it may "cast doubt on the generalizability of several tenets of psychosocial health and health disparities," said Ruiz.

He also sounded a caution: Hispanic longevity and health outcomes are relatively good news, but their health is not optimal and the risk factors in their lives cannot be ignored. The field must not decide that "Hispanic health is better, so let's focus on somebody else," urged Ruiz.

Few studies have actually measured cultural values and related them to objective physical health indicators, leading Ruiz to characterize the sociocultural hypothesis for Hispanic health advantages as "promising yet untested." More research can advance understanding of how resilience works, test ideas in targeted interventions, and guide studies of resilience in other underserved populations. This, he said, "may be where some answers lie and where we can push the field to make the next advance."

> *The emerging science of cultural resilience may open the next wave of health contribution opportunities with implications for all. —John M. Ruiz*

Mind, Body, Spirit: Native Cultures and Well-Being

Historians and sociologists generally agree that centuries of colonialism, supported by federal policies aimed at destroying Native cultures, undermined the economic, social, and spiritual well-being of Native people.[25] Forcibly removed from their lands and prohibited from practicing their religions and traditions, many tribes were unable to nurture their members and sustain their systems of commerce and trade.

For more than one hundred years, federal legislation authorized the removal of Native children from their homes, placing them in boarding schools with the explicit aim of purging them of their cultures. Severely punished for speaking their language or engaging in other Native traditions, many children returned home years later, disconnected from their families and communities.

The effects of that entire historical trauma endure. Suicide rates among Native youth are 2.5 times higher than the national average, and Native youth are five times more likely than white youth to be in the criminal justice system. More than 80 percent of Native adults report having experienced violence in their lives.[26]

Yet Native cultures, traditions, and values have managed to survive decades of official and sustained attempts to destroy them. Almost 6.8 million American Indians and Native Alaskans live in the United States, including people of mixed ancestry who identify as Native.[27] They belong to 573 federally recognized tribes in 35 states.[28] About 22 percent live on one of the approximately 326 federally recognized reservations, and 60 percent live in metropolitan areas.[29]

Their world-view remains unique in many ways. In distinguishing Native and Western cultures, a report prepared for *Native Americans in Philanthropy*[30] observes that Native people "see their responsibility as living in harmonious and balanced relation with all creation, including other tribes and racial/ethnic communities. In contrast, Western Europeans understand the world and the meaning of life in terms of history and tend to orient their life towards the future, towards goals, destiny, and final purpose."

Native American Connections

Diana Yazzie Devine has worked with Native people since a 1972 undergraduate internship took her to the Ojibwe community in northern Wisconsin. Subsequent travels landed her in Arizona, where in 1979 she was introduced to Indian Rehabilitation, a new residential addiction treatment facility in Phoenix, by a member of its board of directors.

Back then, the agency had only two employees, and Yazzie Devine agreed to help out until a leader could be hired. That was more than 39 years ago, and she has served as its only president and chief executive officer ever since. The agency—now called Native American Connections—has 180 employees and annual income of more than $15 million, with $34 million in total assets as of 2017.

Native American Connections offers a unique blend of Native and western housing, clinical, psychological, and spiritual experiences to help both Native and non-Native participants heal and thrive. From the outset, Yazzie Devine understood that Native values would guide the agency. "Our model then, and our model now, is three interlocking circles—a healthy mind, a healthy body, and a healthy spirit," she said. "That's what people call wellness today."

> *Native American traditional healing practices anchor evidence-based practices to foster an empowering and supportive environment; creating a pathway to hope, wellness, and an improved quality of life. —Native American Connections*

The following highlighted programs are just a sample of the many offerings at Native American Connections, all anchored in Native tradition and culture.

Behavioral Health Services

Native American Connections delivers a range of residential and outpatient behavioral programs for children, teens, young adults, and adults. These are grounded in Native tradition while also incorporating best practices endorsed by the Substance Abuse and Mental Health Services Administration (SAMHSA). The intent is to draw on sound evidence and adhere to regulations, but also to ensure that cultural identity becomes a building block of healing.

About 360 people participate in one of the agency's treatment programs every day; about 65 percent of those participants are Native. Programs, including the two described here, are supported by a mix of federal, state, and tribal agencies and by private insurance. Another 50-bed residential treatment facility is under development.

The Patina Wellness Center

This 70-bed center provides residential substance use treatment focused on integrating mind, body, and spirit. It serves men and women, including parents who bring their children. Participants attend life skills and health education classes, workforce development activities, and other skill-building efforts. The center also provides computers, wellness checks, alternative healing practices, art therapy, and on-site childcare for children up to 5 years of age.

Services draw on the approach used at the Hazelden Betty Ford Foundation, a well-regarded treatment system, but "we flipped the curriculum to be sure the core services are about healing the spirit," Yazzie Devine said. This contrasts with most hospital-based treatment programs, where people "generally don't get spiritual healing from trauma and connections to community and self," she noted.

Morning sessions at the center feature recovery education and life skills training. In the afternoon, participants engage in Native practices, including sweat lodges, talking circles, and drumming (all described below). They create Native crafts, draw family trees, and learn about their tribal histories and traditions. "We learn one set of things in the morning and apply those learnings through a Native tradition in the afternoon," Yazzie Devine said.

Transition to Independence

While attending one of the intensive outpatient treatment programs offered by Native American Connections, participants have an opportunity to live in Pendleton Court (for women) or Indian Rehabilitation (for men) as a first step toward independent living. Supported by a live-in recovery coach, residents become part of the transitional community, contributing to household chores and engaging in other shared activities. As they progress toward self-sufficiency, residents start to assume costs of food and other basic needs.

Affordable Housing in Native Style

Yazzie Devine considers Native American Connections' housing services "the foundation for supporting people in their recovery, building family stability, and promoting community wellness." The agency develops, owns, and operates 743 units (with 194 more in development), housing more than 1,100 people in several locations throughout Phoenix. Approximately 40 percent of residents are Native. Housing development and subsidies are supported by rental income, tax credits, vouchers for veteran services, the Department of Housing and Urban Development, and state and city funds.

The agency's housing developments bring traditional Native culture into modern brick-and-mortar settings. Facades use earth-tone colors that blend with desert geography. Expansive windows allow an abundance of natural light into apartments. Plantings and landscaping reflect Arizona's natural terrain and climate.

Colorful common areas encourage community and neighborly relationships. The units are sited in upscale and mixed-income residential and commercial neighborhoods that provide residents with a vibrant urban living experience. One complex, Devine Legacy, is the first housing community in Arizona to receive Leadership in Energy and Environmental Design (LEED) Platinum designation, the highest possible level.[31]

Affordable housing is available for families, older adults, people with disabilities, chronically homeless men and women, and homeless youth. When necessary, residents receive support to ensure they pay their rent, maintain their homes, engage with one another, and enjoy the benefits of independent living. Residential options include:

- **Permanent supportive housing:** Five supportive housing complexes provide housing and on- and off-site services for low-income people who have been chronically homeless and need extra medical, social, and life skills (e.g., budgeting) help to live independently. Supportive housing allows staff to "really see the human being and not just the person other people didn't want around," Yazzie Devine said. The complexes provide more than 275 furnished and unfurnished studio and one-bedroom units.
- **Permanent affordable housing:** Seven complexes provide more than 400 affordable rental units for working low- and moderate-income individuals and families, including two for older adults. Units range from studios to

four-bedroom units. An additional complex is slated to open at the end of 2019.

- **HomeBase:** This 25-bed residence for homeless youth ages 18 to 24 provides young people with a safe place to live off the streets. Residents can attend high school equivalency or college readiness classes, and receive help to find jobs, manage their finances, and participate in activities that promote wellness.

The Phoenix Indian School Visitor Center

The Phoenix Indian Boarding School, located on 160 acres in central Phoenix, housed Native children from 1891 to 1990. When it closed, the property became a city park, but "the Native community was completely left out" of the planning, said Yazzie Devine.

Times began to change, with Native people asserting their rights to respect and a place at the table, and public officials recognizing the importance of their contributions. Almost 30 years after the boarding school closed its doors, and after extensive negotiations between Native American Connections, the city of Phoenix, and other public and private partners, the school reopened in 2017 as the Phoenix Indian School Visitor Center. It features conference space, a commercial kitchen, tribal meeting space, classes, and an exhibit space. Native American Connections operates the center.

Native Ceremonies Promote Healing

Native practices and ceremonies are infused into all of the activities and services delivered at Native American Connections, contributing to the resurgence of Native culture. "Ceremonies and culture are so integrated into tribal life," said Yazzie Devine, explaining why it is meaningful to rekindle that history. "Those are healing practices that over time bring the long-lasting connections to the community that help wellness far beyond the service delivery system."

Sweat Lodges

The Sweat Lodge, representing the womb of Mother Earth, is a sacred space to ask for healing, forgiveness, hope, and vision; and to give thanks and to ask for anything else you might need on your journey. —Native American Connections

Sweat lodges are an ancient purification ceremony for prayer and healing. Preparing for the ceremony is considered an honor and undertaken with care. It begins with cleaning and arranging the grounds, building and tending the fire, and "dressing" the lodge to get it ready. Lodges themselves are circular or oblong domes built with natural material covered with blankets or animal skins. Water is poured over heated stones placed in the center of the lodge, creating steam.

A sweat leader—an elder who knows the tribe's language, songs, and traditions—guides members in traditional prayer and song, and in personal expression. Held weekly, sweat lodges are a core part of Native American Connections' residential and outpatient treatment.

Talking Circles

In talking circles, participants learn to speak "from a place of sincerity and truth-fulness," said Yazzie Devine. A traditional practitioner opens with a prayer or story. Following ancient practices handed down from elders, participants sit in a circle in a circular room, listen deeply, and then speak from their hearts. Some purify, or "smudge," themselves with smoke from burning herbs. A feather or talking stick is passed around the circle in a "sunwise" direction, inviting and en-couraging participants as they hold it, to speak without interruption, criticism, or judgment.

Drumming

Drums are central to Native celebrations, ceremonies, and talking circles. To Native peoples, they represent the heartbeat of Mother Earth, who speaks through the drum and the drummer to reunite the physical and mental being with the spiritual self. Drums are considered sacred objects, entrusted only to designated keepers. Their rhythms, whether meditative or energetic, promote self-expression through dance and movement. People "have to approach the drum in a healthy way, with mind, body, and spirit," said Yazzie Devine. Rather than simply helping people stop using substances, "we are creating a lifestyle and a pathway back into the community through drumming."

Drumming benefits non-Native people as well. Yazzie Devine remembers "flowing tears" coming from a young man who had struggled with metham-phetamine addiction when he joined a drumming ceremony within a talking circle. The young man released "every emotion he had suppressed," she recalled, still moved by the memory. The man went on to work with Native American Connections for seven years. "Native ceremonies can reach people at a different level" than people expect or than is typical of other treatment protocols, said Yazzie Devine.

Circles of Strength

Over one weekend each month, a circle of strength brings families together in a two-day facilitated experience in which people attending treatment and their families join in a program of education, skills building, and family-centered problem-solving. They also engage together in traditional Native arts, music, and other cultural activities. The goal is to repair family ties that often fray when a family member uses substances. The weekend concludes with a talking circle. Between 30 and 50 people participate in a circle of strength each month.

Native Values, Robert Wood Johnson Foundation's Vision, and the Pull of the Past

Long before the term "Culture of Health" was coined, Native values reflected many of its goals. The Native view of life as cyclical finds expression in the circle of equity that surrounds the Culture of Health described by the Robert Wood Johnson Foundation (RWJF). The importance of harmony, family, and community is echoed in the goals and values of RWJF's Action Areas. The language that informs a Culture of Health—equity, well-being, integration, and community—patterns Native idioms that describe the mind, body, and spirit as inseparable; that honor the healing power of community; and that demonstrate respect for all life—people, animals, and the earth itself.

A Final Word

The stories of the Hispanic paradox and the healing power of Native traditions speak to the role of culture as a force for well-being. Ruiz delivers evidence that *familismo, simpatico,* and *respeto* can foster resilience and health, even in the face of disproportionate risk. Yazzie Devine explains how strong cultural traditions can be infused into evidence-based programs to promote harmony and healing.

Each of these groups continues to face discrimination and disproportionately high rates of poverty, but the cultural assets that give them strength are critical buffers against the marginalizing forces of inequality. Highlighting those assets also helps to shift the narrative as it informs mainstream culture, which has traditionally overlooked those who have been excluded from it. A shared understanding of the contributions and values of other cultures opens the doors wider to improving the health outcomes of people from all backgrounds.

A Note About Language

Words matter when we describe a culture, race, ethnic group, population, or gender. In a pluralistic society, decisions about language must be made intentionally, and with respect. Indeed, discussions about language, and the meanings underlying it, might be first steps in bridging divides among people who might feel inappropriately labeled or stereotyped by terms others perceive as innocuous.

The terminologies sometimes used to describe the groups featured in this chapter alone suggest the complexity of the issue:

People with ancestors from Spanish-speaking countries may prefer to be called brown, Hispanic, Latina/o, Chicana/o, and most recently, Latinx. Which words should be used, and when?

Indigenous peoples may prefer Native American, American Indian, First Nation, or Native, or the name of their tribe. In which situations should which word be used?

People with African or West Indian ancestors may choose black, African American, West Indian, or person of color. Is one preferable, or does the context matter most?

People with European ancestors might consider themselves white, Caucasian, or European American. Which is most appropriate, and when?

There is no right answer to any of these questions, because no single term captures an entire group in all its diversity and preferences. Certainly, no one person can represent or speak for everyone who shares a similar cultural background.

The contributors to this chapter were asked to speak only on behalf of their work, drawing from their research and experiences. The chapter uses "Hispanic" because that term is widely used in Census and other data. It uses "Native American Connections" when referring to the organization of that name, and "Native" in other contexts because Diana Yazzie Devine uses that term in presentations and conversations. These were deliberate choices, thoughtfully made, but by no means the only options available.

How Media Shapes the Public Discourse and Influences Health

Erika Franklin Fowler, PhD, MA, Associate Professor, Department of Government and Co-Director, Wesleyan Media Project, Wesleyan University

Sarah Gollust, PhD, Associate Professor, Division of Health Policy and Management, School of Public Health, University of Minnesota

Nat Gyenes, MPH, Senior Program Manager, Meedan; Research Affiliate, Berkman Klein Center for Internet & Society, Harvard University

Can lemons cure AIDS? That became a tantalizing teaser headline used in multiple stories after Australian researchers suggested at an International Society of Spermatology meeting that a certain concentration of lemon-juice solution seemed to kill HIV in a laboratory petri dish.

Erika Franklin Fowler uncovered that claim in her 2002 review of health coverage on local television news, conducted with researchers from the University of Wisconsin and the University of Michigan. The problem with that kind of reporting, of course, is that it provides no contextual information (e.g., failing to indicate when research is in its most preliminary phase, or conducted in the laboratory, rather than in humans). Sometimes the distortion is much worse. One story about the purported lemon-juice cure claimed it could be used in place of "costly HIV medications." Fowler's analysis revealed other "egregious errors" that could do harm as well, and she noted that among almost 1,400 stories covering various diseases, "few gave recommendations, cited specific data sources or discussed prevalence of the health conditions" being described.[1]

All of that suggests the news media operate far from the ideal of conveying accurate and actionable information about the many dimensions of health, informing conversation, influencing policy, and making the Culture of Health normative. In today's media landscape, which is as broad and diverse as the

Culture of Health in Practice, Alonzo L. Plough. Oxford University Press (2020) © Robert Wood Johnson Foundation
DOI: 10.1093/oso/9780190071400.001.0001

audiences who watch, read, tweet, or share it, misinformation and bias are proliferating as complex issues are oversimplified and facts distorted.

News coverage is also shaped by economic realities. Save for a handful of public broadcasting stations, virtually all media platforms operate in a for-profit milieu and seldom view education as their paramount function. No matter how dedicated their editorial staff, advertising sustains and is likely to influence content, and the importance of attracting consumers largely determines the topics and how they are positioned. And that framework doesn't even consider the role of entertainment media, which makes no claim at all to be a purveyor of facts, but nonetheless serves as a source of information, sometimes a primary source, for a vast populace.

The angle from which current events are covered is another important characteristic of media influence, reflecting or shifting the public discourse and swaying the responses that gain traction. Stories that frame obesity as a personal responsibility, for example, can drive public support for one set of policies, while emphasizing the influence of structural forces, such as government regulation and industry advertising, builds interest in others.

For the news media to help build a Culture of Health, we need to understand how it works, what it does, and how it can be used for widespread benefit. Four contributors to this chapter help do just that. Erika Franklin Fowler and Sarah Gollust outline the core functions of media in society, elaborating on its role as a tool for socialization, agenda setting, investigation, information, framing, and persuasion. Nat Gyenes explores the diffuse media networks that often make it difficult for public health to get its message out. Finally, in a Spotlight profile, Jennifer Harris takes a look at how the food industry markets unhealthy products to black and Latino youth.

The Many Roles of Media

In a stage-setting question at the media breakout session of the 2018 *Sharing Knowledge* conference, Erika Franklin Fowler asked the audience, "What is one word that comes to mind when you think about the media's role in society?" The varied answers—inflame, invasive, powerful, propaganda, sense-making, overwhelming, perverse, polarization, culture, and controversy—suggest the many ways in which media infiltrate our lives. Fowler and Sarah Gollust touched on some of those characteristics as they described the key functions of media.

Socialization

Media help to cultivate and convey community beliefs and norms. "Media convey values, and provide important inroads for what we as a society value," said Fowler. In an *Annual Review of Public Health* article, Fowler, Gollust, and a colleague at Cornell University elaborated on the public health implications of the socialization role through the lens of television news.[2]

"TV news can promote health-improving norms, enhance citizens' sense of community and social connectedness and increase their civic participation," they wrote. But exposure can also shift viewer perceptions to align with the ways in which television portrays reality. For example, local news disproportionately features crime stories, and people who watch it more frequently are more likely to perceive crime as a significant social problem.

Agenda-Setting

Another very powerful function of media is to set the agenda. Given the limited attention span of policymakers and the public at large, issues that draw media coverage are more likely to gain a spot in the public square. "In the classic agenda-setting framework, media don't tell us what to think, but they tell us what to think about," Fowler said. "If the media are focused on a given issue, it becomes harder for policymakers to ignore it."

The reverse is also true: Topics that don't make it onto the media agenda are less likely to gain traction among policymakers or become a topic of concern among the general public. From that perspective, media's tendency to bypass nuanced analyses of complex social challenges in favor of hot-button issues has consequences. When it comes to health, for example, media are more likely to cover health care than to look closely at the social determinants of health.

The media's limited perception of what belongs on the agenda is evident in the thin coverage of health equity, the lens through which the Robert Wood Johnson Foundation does so much of its work. A 2009 analysis of almost seven hundred articles from 19 newspapers found that 87 percent of them did not mention disparities in their discussions of type 2 diabetes.[3] A more recent study of four local New England newspapers was even more disappointing, revealing that just 3 percent of 650 health stories mentioned either disparities or social determinants of health.[4]

Many factors may explain the gap. "You can dig deep into structural inequities embedded in both media and academia to identify reasons why equity in health is not top of mind for journalists," observed Gollust. With structural racism at the root of many equity challenges, reporters may be deterred by the complexity of the subject, reluctant to take it on before an audience they presume (perhaps inappropriately) to be primarily white, or they may be discouraged by the reality that inequities are an enduring problem, not the novel development they generally prefer to cover.

We need to see what's on the agenda, and of course, what's not. What doesn't even make it onto the agenda? —Sarah Gollust

Investigating and Informing

Through their investigative role, and as information-sharing vehicles, media can illuminate topics that might otherwise remain invisible, again helping to determine what rises to the level of widely shared awareness.

That is evident in a survey conducted by the Kaiser Family Foundation that assessed how people learned about the Affordable Care Act (ACA).[5] A plurality of respondents (44%) said their impression was based mainly on television, radio, and newspapers, compared to 23 percent who got their information from personal experience and 18 percent who got it from family and friends. Fowler and Gollust linked television viewer data to this survey information and found that those with higher levels of exposure to local ACA news coverage were more likely to say they had enough information about it.[6]

We observed a relationship between volume of media exposure and this knowledge-related outcome. That helps to explain why it is critically important that we understand what messages the media is sending the public about health policy issues. —Sarah Gollust

The extent of media consumption can also inform the public's health and health care decision-making. For example, one study conducted by Gollust, Fowler, and their colleagues found that counties in which the audience had greater exposure to advertising from both public and private health insurers were more likely to see uninsured rates drop and Medicaid coverage increase.[7]

Here, too, media's hold on its audience is a double-edged sword, given its potential to offer both misinformation and disinformation. Misinformation can result from unintentional errors or a poor translation of complex facts, while disinformation is the intentional spread of something known to be false. Overplaying the medical significance of a new drug that has been tested only on a small number of animals is one example of misinformation, while the accusation that the Affordable Care Act intended to fund "death panels" under Medicare is disinformation promoted for ideological reasons.

Even if the information itself is accurate, the angle of coverage or the repetition of a story can distort viewer perception, or result in misperceptions of disease risk. The way in which many people have come to view potential carcinogens offers one example of this. "Because of the rapidity with which local news presents on new studies, new associations, new epidemiological findings, consumers actually have more fatalistic views about cancer," said Gollust. "They believe that everything causes cancer."[8, 9]

Framing

Media play an important framing role, with implications for how societal challenges are analyzed and addressed. "The media frame issues so as to emphasize particular causes, solutions, and policy approaches," said Gollust. "And that framing can also invite the public to make moral assessments of those health and social issues." For example, whether opioid use is presented as an individual failing, a crime, or a medical issue helps determine the nature of the public debate, the extent of the stigma associated with it, and ultimately the policies put in place to address it.[10]

Industry responsibility for public health challenges has increasingly become part of the competitive nature of frames in public health discourse. Long a feature of the tobacco control debate, the industry role has more recently entered discussions about sugar-sweetened beverage taxes. Although research indicates that positioning industry as the "villain" in the story promotes overall support for the tax, that strategy also may prompt a backlash, especially among those who are predisposed to oppose such taxes.[11]

Persuasion

Yet another core function of media is to be persuasive. Advertising—the lifeblood of most media—is an obvious example. In 2016, food companies alone spent $13.5 billion to advertise food, beverages, and restaurants, with just 50 companies accounting for more than 70 percent of that spending.[12] To put that in context, the entire budget for chronic disease prevention and health promotion at the Centers for Disease Control and Prevention (CDC) is less than $1.2 billion.[13] (Although food advertising reaches all sociodemographic groups, unhealthy beverages and snacks are disproportionately marketed to young people of color, with implications that are explored more fully in the Chapter 2 Spotlight: "Media Marketing to Minority Youth.")

Commentators, bloggers, and opinion writers on numerous traditional and social media platforms also act as persuaders. With ever-sharper political lines being drawn in the United States, the result is that different media are reaching different audiences, with messages that often promote particular viewpoints or policy actions and tend to reinforce existing biases and beliefs.

The Media Landscape Today

The environment in which these media functions are performed is evolving rapidly, with broad societal implications. As information sources multiply, they are increasingly varied in tone and focus, and that heterogeneity makes it harder to set a collective agenda.

In the broadcasting era, news production was more centralized, with morning newspapers and nightly television serving as the primary sources of highly trusted and widely shared information. But today, messengers battle one another for attention, across platforms and on multiple programs in the same time slot. Fierce competition, changes to funding structures, and cuts to dedicated health reporting have altered the landscape, forcing reporters with less expertise in health and less time to connect with knowledgeable sources to produce stories around the clock on tighter budgets.

The pace of the reporting, in particular the pressure to break news, makes it especially difficult to provide the context necessary to help audiences appreciate, say, the significance of a new finding or the distinction between association and causality. "The news is always going to look for the novelty and simplicity in presentation, which makes it hard to convey nuances," Fowler said. As a result, the art of distilling and disseminating complex ideas, without inaccuracy or exaggeration, is at risk.

> *If you think about trying to design a headline that gets people to click on it, it might look very different than if you are trying to accurately reflect the content. We know what sort of news tends to draw eyeballs. —Erika Franklin Fowler*

Early messaging on the ACA demonstrates just how competitive the media environment has become. On television alone, at least four sets of messengers were communicating with the public during the first open-enrollment period of the health insurance marketplace: partisan actors in campaign advertising railing against a "government takeover" of health care, local news broadcasters offering information about access to ACA-related benefits or discussing the latest partisan bickering on the subject, state-based exchanges calling attention to the availability of coverage, and private insurers trying to attract consumers to their plans.

"That gives you a sense of the different types of messaging that occur inside just one medium," said Fowler. "And of course in this more fragmented environment, there are lots of other places to go for ACA-related information. How this all translates into citizen knowledge and opinion can be challenging to sort out."

Deep polarization adds to the noise, with audiences able to "select the source of information that is more likely to cohere with their world-view," she added. "That can have great benefits because it allows for tailoring and ease of finding information they care about, but it can also allow people to filter information through their own mind-set. In the health context, that can be very concerning."

In this splintered environment, the voices of independent journalists are just one part of a much larger cast. Corporations, government entities, institutions, think tanks, and political partisans are also trying to reach the public, through both the news media and more direct communication pathways.

Journalists write and frame stories, but they're not the only actors here. It's very simplistic to think about a news story as though that is the only infor- mation consumers will hear and that it will impact the public in some kind of monolithic way. —Erika Franklin Fowler

"Audiences have multiple exposures to health information," said Gollust, reinforcing the theme. "They may get health information from best friends or doctors or news or advertisements. Before a message reaches them, they may already be both pre-exposed and predisposed to accept or reject the message. Their prior exposure and their attitudinal and ideological predispositions shape the way they respond."

Television remains the primary source of news for many Americans, with local stations drawing the largest audiences. Coverage that is geographically defined—as is the case with local TV news—has the potential to promote a shared understanding of common regional problems, but that opportunity too often is subsumed by an emphasis on political squabbles. Further, local television stations are vulnerable to changes in ownership, which can lead to homogeniza- tion of content, rather than to promoting variation across geographic regions.[14]

In a study published in the *American Journal of Public Health*, for example, researchers looked at local television news stories about the ACA during its early rollout (October 1, 2013–April 19, 2014).[15] More than half (55%) of the stories presented political disagreements, framing ACA implementation as a matter of wins and losses—what Gollust called "horse race coverage." One-third of the stories were about website failures, and 27 percent reported on the number of enrollees to date. The major policy tools of the ACA—Medicaid expansion and premium subsidies—were each cited just 7 percent of the time. "The news likes to cover politics, controversy, and conflict," continued Gollust.

Audiences seem to like that emphasis as well. "Audiences have always demanded to be entertained and drawn into the conflicts of the day," she noted. In their quest for clicks, media look for provocative, even sensational, language, especially in their headlines and sometimes at the price of rigor.

Media Networks: Diffuse and Isolated

Building on this analysis of media's many functions, Nat Gyenes looked at the diffusion of online health information, which is rapidly gaining viewership, in line with broader trends. In 2016, 57 percent of U.S. adults were "often" getting news of all sorts from television, according to the Pew Center; two years later, that figure had fallen to 49 percent. Online sources—news websites and social media—filled most of the gap, rising from 38 percent in 2016 to 43 percent in 2018. Television remains dominant primarily among older audiences, suggesting that over time this balance will continue to shift.[16]

Gyenes, too, opened her presentation at the *Sharing Knowledge* media breakout session with a question to the audience: "Where do you get your health information?" Although some people indicated they rely on specific, credible websites, the most common response was: "through a Google search." Pleading guilty to seeking some of her own medical information that way, Gyenes acknowledged, "We look for symptoms in Google. We don't *necessarily* consult the CDC's website when we have the flu."

That an informed public health group sometimes uses potentially unreliable sources highlights another hazard of rapidly proliferating media. An online search for "breast cancer and diet" quickly uncovers a newspaper article about the role of dairy products in fueling tumors and a website that definitively identifies sugar as the primary culprit. Both assertions have a weak scientific basis, but lots of popular support. With the broad access that consumers have to blogs, Facebook groups, and countless other social resources, they can readily bypass traditional medical expertise and go straight to their peers to discuss symptoms and exchange treatment ideas.

Some of these misleading ideas tend to travel like an infectious disease, writes Gyenes in the *Atlantic*:[17]

> We know that memes—whether about cute animals or health-related misinformation—spread like viruses: mutating, shifting, and adapting rapidly until one idea finds an optimal form and spreads quickly. What we have yet to develop are effective ways to identify, test, and vaccinate against these misinfo-memes. —Nat Gyenes

The siloed nature of present-day media presents further challenges because it "allows people the opportunity to craft news environments that reflect and reinforce their attitudes and biases," writes Brian Weeks in an essay in the compendium *Misinformation and Mass Audiences*.[18] Rather than breaking down walls, our media selections allow us to remain comfortably within information bubbles of our own choosing.

Although these bubbles may reflect a singular point of view, they are unlikely to be confined to a solitary source. A compelling story tends to travel through multiple outlets, with coverage in one setting prompting further coverage of the same development in other formats.

"Narratives transfer from journal articles through to news articles or TV programs and end up traveling in networks," explained Gyenes. "These networks, which provide information that shapes our perception of norms, can often be quite isolated from one another.

"In a sense, public health is its own information network," Gyenes said. Research from the Media Lab at the Massachusetts Institute of Technology (MIT) indicates that institutions such as the CDC, the World Health Organization, schools of public health at leading universities such as Harvard and Johns Hopkins, and RWJF all tend to use the same terminology and to cite one another.[19] They are part of a network accustomed to sharing a unique language, speaking comfortably about epidemiology, statistics, intersectionality, and social determinants of health with colleagues and in peer-reviewed articles.

In many cases, however, that cluster of information sources "is not linked effectively to the rest of the media network," Gyenes pointed out, an assertion that Gollust and colleagues affirmed in one of their studies. Their work found that only 4 percent of news stories covering the ACA's rollout actually cited findings from foundations, think tanks, or academics. Sources with a political affiliation—including President Barack Obama, federal agency staff, and Republican and Democratic public officials—were far more common.[20]

That has to change if a Culture of Health is to take hold, but the efforts of public health experts to share information with the public through third parties, including traditional and online media, often fall flat. "It turns out that it is really hard to translate our messages," observed Gyenes.

"We forget that we as public health professionals are communicating in a language that we were forced to learn—the language of statistics and epidemiology, and of methodologies that are used to distinguish between causality and correlation. And we are sharing information using a language with others who may not have learned it yet. Our patterns of sharing information don't diffuse out to the rest of the digital information network."

A partisan bent to language choices can be a potent impediment to consensus. Gyenes reported on an evaluation of news media sorted by political leaning, which found that although common terminology generally is used in covering child health, obesity, education, cancer, and overdoses, terminology differed when other topics were being discussed:[21]

- **Wellness and well-being:** Left-leaning media tend to speak about "wellness" while right-leaning sources more frequently use the term "well-being."

- **Environmental health:** The left focuses on climate change and its impacts, while right-leaning media tend to talk about interactions with the built environment, diet, and exercise.
- **Public health strategies:** There is something of an "us-versus-them" theme on the left, with words like "empathy" and "advocate" used frequently; on the right, the language of teamwork and collaboration appear more often.
- **New health information:** Significant differences emerge in how the scientific method is covered. While left-leaning sources use terms such as "research" and "researchers" to suggest a body of knowledge, the right often refers to "studies," which can be individual findings that are not necessarily aligned with a larger set of accumulating knowledge.

Gyenes suggested that highlighting a single study, rather than referencing a full body of research, makes it easier to change, and possibly distort, a narrative. Generalizing from one set of findings ignores possible design limitations, methodological flaws, and the likelihood that the study was intended to examine a narrow circumstance or population. "That is one of our leads when we are trying to understand the spread of health misinformation," she said.

Media coverage of vaccines is an example of why language matters. As misinformation about the relationship between vaccines and adverse health effects spreads within a network, it tends to normalize the decision to avoid vaccinations. From their own silo, public health authorities lambast that tendency, using terms like "pro-vaccination" and "anti-vaccination," despite research that reveals them to be highly polarizing; references to "vaccine-confident" and "vaccine-hesitant" communities are seen as less judgmental.

"Because of our difficulties in creating a common understanding and language, and not being able to connect narratives beyond our own public health information community to the broader information ecosystem, some current attempts to combat health misinformation don't really work," Gyenes warned.

Digging deeper into the problem, she references research conducted on Twitter at MIT's Media Lab, which found a faster diffusion of falsehoods than truth in its study sample.[22] Falsehoods may be shared because they confirm an existing view, or as a form of entertainment or "cheerleading," not necessarily because they are assumed to be accurate. That, however, does little to weaken their influence.

Many reasons account for the fragmentation of the media ecosystem and the resulting self-selection of audiences into discrete and disconnected networks. Regardless of the package of causes, however, these are unquestionably significant impediments to the shared understanding needed to shift the societal narrative toward a Culture of Health.

Using Media to Build a Culture of Health

Given media's capacity to help infuse a health focus across society, and the importance of accurate and reasoned arguments to drive policy discussions, advocates of a Culture of Health need to become more strategic in their communication. How can public health professionals move beyond their familiar silos to work effectively with media? How can they frame complex information in language that resonates with a wide audience? Is a shared agenda even possible when so many health-related discussions are divisive?

The public health community can help provide some of the answers by becoming more engaged in the public debate. Fowler advised researchers and advocates to introduce themselves to journalists as sources of in-depth health information and to invest in building relationships. "Reach out, provide yourself as a resource, and talk about the resources journalists can link to or that can offer additional information to their audiences," she urged.

> *Collaborations between news organizations and academic or public health organizations and science communicators can be very fruitful. Scholars and science communicators can help educate all parties involved. —Erika Franklin Fowler*

Some institutions already employ staff with specific expertise in outreach both to the media and to advocates. "As a scientist, I don't know how to speak their language, but we have people who do," commented Jennifer Harris, referring to the University of Connecticut's Rudd Center for Food Policy and Obesity. "They are the bridge between our research and those who use it."

Gollust proposed the idea of creating organizations outside academia that are specifically charged with developing evidence-based syntheses and communicating health-related information. Offering communications training to researchers, including insights into the constraints of the current media environment, is another avenue worth exploring.

She also suggested that funders require dissemination planning in their grants to ensure that scholars start thinking early in their study design about how best to craft resonant messages. "We need to further engrain the concepts of designing for dissemination at the start of health research projects," Gollust said.

In the digital space, identifying the online networks to which audiences are connected is key. "We can look at these online networks and figure out how and who we are trying to target, and adapt our language" to reach them, advised Gyenes. She also underscored the need for broader outreach to bloggers,

YouTube celebrities, and other social media thought leaders who have significant followings.

> *We should encourage the public health community to develop frames that reflect and transmit its values to the broader society.* —Nat Gyenes

To help push beyond their silos, researchers need to expand the sources of the links they embed into digital media content ("in-linking"). Links to concise, relatable explanatory materials can overcome knowledge gaps and provide needed context and perspective. "If public health information authorities could engage in better in-linking practices and encourage journalists who are talking about our content to link back to our reports, it could potentially reduce misinformation," urged Gyenes.

The public health community needs to become better at storytelling. Narratives are a useful tool for discussing technical issues in comprehensible language, and for reducing the stigma that is a well-established barrier to optimal public health practice. Gollust emphasized that "really rich narratives, ones that are sympathetic and identify and situate individuals within their social/structural context" are a way to introduce audiences to real people dealing with issues that tend to be stigmatized, such as substance use disorder, mental illness, and obesity.

Promoting health and media literacy, starting in the early years of school, is another strategy to foster informed discussion and prudent decision-making. But welcome though such training would be, it does not substitute for accurate, actionable information, presented in language that laypeople can understand at any stage of their lives.

Gyenes offered an anecdote to underscore the importance of knowledge translation. In a casual conversation, her taxi driver mentioned getting much of his health information from the television personality Dr. Phil. Gyenes delicately suggested he might look to other resources instead, but when the driver asked, "Like who?" she found that she had nothing to suggest.

"I could name foundations, I could highlight reports, I could reference academic institutions that are doing some really incredible intersectional work," she said, while recognizing that these were unlikely to grab his attention.

> *There isn't a forward-thinking, leading public health information authority that's entertaining and interesting and can cross these partisanship boundaries.* —Nat Gyenes

Filling that gap, she concluded, might be something worth adding to our to-do list.

A Final Word

The importance of accurate information takes on increasing urgency in a politically fractured era, especially at a time when inequity impedes a Culture of Health. As media sources multiply, each targeting a narrow band of audience, it is easier than ever to oversell a finding, confuse or distort a fact, or divide a people.

"Everyone is entitled to his own opinion, but not to his own facts," said Senator Daniel Patrick Moynihan decades ago. Although that point of view is being challenged as never before, it suggests a guardrail that urgently needs to be reinforced.

That media should provide a baseline of shared knowledge—offering citizens a nuanced perspective on issues relevant to their lives—might seem like an antiquated concept in today's society. But for all of its flaws and challenges, from the partisan schisms within its ranks to the pressures of advertising, media remains a positive force for building a Culture of Health and the equity agenda that makes it possible. Deconstructing its many roles—socialization and agenda-setting, informing and investigating, persuading and framing—is a critical step toward broadening the base of astute news consumers.

Chapter 2 Spotlight: Media Marketing to Minority Youth

Jennifer Harris, PhD, MBA, Rudd Center for Food Policy and Obesity, University of Connecticut

Jennifer Harris probed media's role as a persuader, focusing her analyses on how food advertisers target black and Latino/a youth with the marketing of unhealthy products. "Food advertising contributes to health disparities and makes it much more difficult for us to encourage a Culture of Health," she argued.

Carefully placed TV ads, marketing in low-income minority communities, and buying good will through philanthropy and the sponsorship of sports and music events are all industry strategies to promote foods high in fat, sugar, and salt. "The least healthy products are the ones that are targeted most to these communities," Harris said. Hershey, Mars, PepsiCo, and Wendy's are among the companies that invest a high proportion of their total TV ad budget specifically in the black youth market.[1] Kraft Foods, Mars, and McDonald's take particular aim at Hispanic young people.[2]

On average, black teens see more than twice as many TV ads as white youth for candy, sugar-sweetened beverages, and snacks—almost 10 a day, according to Nielsen tallies.[3] And Hispanic children and teens are more likely than whites to visit food company websites that target young people with unhealthy food, such as Chuck E. Cheese and Froot Loops.[4] The impact is intensified by the fact that black and Latino youth are also exposed to disproportionately more unhealthy food marketing in their communities, so they get a double dose of exposure.

Advertisers try to convey the message that "their products are fun and cool and exciting," pointed out Harris, and an online survey indicates that across racial and ethnic groups, teens generally agree with this characterization. Research has also shown that black and Hispanic youth follow an average of almost five different food brands on social media (white, non-Hispanics follow 3.6 brands).[5]

A series of focus groups with black and Hispanic teenagers from a low-income area of Hartford, Conn., revealed more about their views of the food brands they identify as most targeted "for someone like me," including Doritos, Gatorade, Pizza Hut, Snickers, and Taco Bell.[6] Typical of their comments:

- "A lot of Latinas would use Coca-Cola and eat a lot of Doritos. Like when there's a party, there's a bag of Doritos."
- "I like the Pop Tarts, Sonic, Twix, and Skittles ads. They're funny. I'll be in a really bad mood and they come on and I start laughing."

Asked how targeted marketing makes them feel, participants were at first overwhelmingly positive about being the locus of advertiser attention:

- "Like in Gatorade commercials, it's always like a football player, it's a black guy, it's encouraging."
- "It makes us feel good because they want everyone to try their products, people from higher or lower social class and from different countries."
- "It makes us feel special, since they are going after us."

But that initial reaction shifted after further conversations. "We discussed the products that they see in their neighborhoods and the types of products where advertisers show people who look like them and they started to get the sense that these products are not good for them," recalled Harris. Those insights fostered an attitudinal change among participants:

- "I feel kind of taken advantage of."
- "I'm not going to go to Wendy's as much as I usually do because I'm not going to give them the satisfaction of causing me to give them my money."
- "They are blanket exploiting the fact that we don't have the resources to go and buy things that taste good and are healthy. We have to limit ourselves to their food."

That shift, said Harris, "really shows that there is an opportunity here to reframe targeted marketing as a social justice issue."

AT HOME, AT SCHOOL, AT WORK

Bringing a Culture of Health to the Places that Surround Our Lives

Ideally, as a Culture of Health moves into the mainstream, it will increasingly become embedded within all of the spaces we occupy—our homes, schools, workplaces, the places where we worship, and the settings in which we gather for recreation and socializing. These places matter because they provide the framework in which children are nurtured, adults are empowered and connected, and communities find and embrace the resources they need to thrive.

For health equity to be possible, the environments in which we spend our days must bring together the elements of a healthy life. Families and individuals can only thrive when these settings are adequately resourced with services that range from health care and banking to housing and recreation; they must be structurally sound, physically secure, and environmentally safe; and they should offer opportunities for engaged community voices and the shared connectivity of family and friends.

The chapters in this section delve deeply into the challenges of bringing the three key pillars of home, school, and work into a Culture of Health. Elements of a fourth and equally vital pillar—play—are suggested in each chapter, where the importance of structured and unstructured play is reflected in the need for parks and community spaces in rural areas, playgrounds and time for recreation in schools, and appropriate health and wellness policies in corporate workplaces.[1]

Chapter 3, "Pathways to Change in Rural America" explores the reputation and reality of the nation's less populated regions, which one in every five people in the United States call home. Too often, the rural designation implies an environment in which poor health and diminished opportunities are the norm. Though the chapter contributors acknowledge the enduring economic, social, and educational inequities that pervade these regions, they are equally invested in capitalizing on the inherent strengths of the rural heritage. Using examples from several Southern rural communities that are among the poorest in the country, yet also offer pockets of hope, the contributors show that it is possible to reshape the narrative of rural living.

Chapter 4, "Linking Education and Health to Support the Whole Child," captures the bidirectional connection between education and health. Healthy children are more successful in school; people with more education are healthier and lead longer lives. But children require a range of supports at home, at school, and in the community to reach their potential—supports that may be woefully lacking in areas of poverty and disadvantage. The chapter's contributors describe the Whole School, Whole Community, Whole Child model, intended to connect education and health by supporting the whole child, and describe a research program designed to advance the broad implementation of that model, especially in under-resourced environments. Also highlighted here is a school-based initiative to encourage healthy eating and active living and to build resilience and foster wellness for school staff and students.

While employers obviously exert tremendous influence on the economic well-being of their employees, it is easy to overlook their role as Culture of Health mediators. Chapter 5, "Employers as Shapers of Health" captures that angle with profiles of four distinct initiatives. Two studies of Fortune 500 companies examine corporate transparency in reporting health-promotion policies and efforts to create healthy work environments and strengthen communities. Another study illustrates the feasibility of stabilizing schedules of low-wage retail workers to benefit workers as well as store sales. The chapter concludes with an example of how one of America's largest employers—the Department of Defense—is building healthy communities through a program that strategically aligns military goals with Culture of Health objectives.

By illustrating the connectivity that drives and sustains a Culture of Health, this section makes it clear that these pillars of a healthy life cannot be siloed or viewed in isolation. Taken together, the elements of home, school, work, and play form a continuum of place where health-generating features are integrated to achieve well-being for individuals and communities alike.

Pathways to Change in Rural America

Ivye L. Allen, PhD, President, Foundation for the Mid South

Mark Drabenstott, Chairman, MarketSquare Inc. and Former Director of the Federal Reserve's Center for the Study of Rural America

Cynthia Mil Duncan, PhD, Professor Emerita of Sociology and Founding Director of the Carsey Institute, University of New Hampshire

Whitney Kimball Coe, Director of National Programs, Center for Rural Strategies

Ed Sivak, Executive Vice President for Policy and Communications, Hope Enterprise Corporation/Hope Credit Union (HOPE)

In the United States, one in every five people live in a rural area. As these approximately 46 million rural residents can attest, small-town America is not just one kind of place. "Rural" cuts across experiences, geography, and sectors, representing such diverse regions as Midwest farming communities, mountain hollows in Appalachia, the indigenous communities of the Southwest, the Central Valley in California, and the segregated communities of the Bible Belt and the Northeast. The rich mix of history, culture, and racial and ethnic populations across rural America is an asset not only to those places but also to our nation.[1] And despite this range of geographic locations, rural communities share many positive touchstones: trademark resilience, interdependence, collaborative spirit, and devotion to family and community.[2]

Today, however, the country is becoming more aware of the conditions in rural America that obstruct the path toward a healthy life. In many rural areas, rising unemployment, shifting demographics, lack of access to good schools and hospitals, high rates of premature death and suicide, and a ruthless opioid epidemic are all well-documented.

At the Robert Wood Johnson Foundation (RWJF), the rural designation has emerged as a health equity focus because "choosing to live in rural America should not present barriers to living a long and healthy life. But too often, it

Culture of Health in Practice, Alonzo L. Plough. Oxford University Press (2020) © Robert Wood Johnson Foundation
DOI: 10.1093/oso/9780190071400.001.0001

does."[3] To enhance health and well-being in rural America, policymakers and advocates must build on the unique challenges, strengths, and opportunities in rural populations. Changes that leverage local resources and strengths to better serve residents are vital, and some of them are surprisingly simple and often community-driven.

This chapter opens with a portrait of rural America, highlighting not only the familiar challenges of equity, race, and poverty but also the unique advantages embedded there. Then, the chapter presents three stories of organizations committed to strengthening rural communities in America, helping the people who live there reshape their own narratives and create pathways to change.

Whitney Kimball Coe of the Center for Rural Strategies explains why she returned to her small-town roots and how forward-looking leaders in rural areas are helping to reshape the rural narrative. Ivye Allen describes the Foundation for the Mid South and the power it has harnessed by investing in human capital through quality education, mentoring, and job training. Ed Sivak reviews Hope Enterprise Corporation/Hope Credit Union (HOPE), a community development financial institution (CDFI) that draws on the foundational strength of anchor institutions such as rural hospitals, banks, and credit unions.

Reshaping the Narrative of the Rural Demise

On December 14, 2018, the *New York Times* ran a lengthy story titled "The Hard Truths of Trying to 'Save' the Rural Economy." The first sentence: "Can rural America be saved?"[4]

Whitney Kimball Coe read the article from her home in Athens, Tenn., quietly seething as she absorbed the by-now predictable, grim litany of problems besetting rural America: aging populations, unemployment, addiction, poverty, poor schools. Five days later—after deliberately taking note of her small town's rich tapestry of neighbors, fellowship, family, work, art, and community—Coe published her blistering and passionate response in a column called "The Rural Heartbeat" on the *Daily Yonder*,[5] a digital newspaper for the rural community.

> *"I don't deny we're fighting some of the demons associated with rural zip codes, but much of these demons are not of our making. They are the result of years and years of disinvestment by the public and private sectors, and of decades of wealth becoming increasingly concentrated in big cities and ivory towers. Yet rural places and small towns still have a heartbeat because people still work, live, and worship in them.*
>
> *"I sure would relish sticking it to The Times and every other self-appointed prophet that presumes to announce the decline of my community or any*

other small town in the United States. They measure our worth in dollars from thousands of miles away, but don't seem to understand that you can't put a price on the way we keep showing up. . . . I'm not ready to cede the richness of this experience—of living in proximity and mutuality with my neighbors—to those who don't have it or don't get it. It's easy to lay bare the demons and deep challenges of far-off places. But it's harder and more rewarding to get close, keep showing up, and be part of the life of a place."

As the director of national programs and coordinator of the Rural Assembly for the Center for Rural Strategies, Coe has made it her life's mission to "keep showing up." And in the process of doing so, she is reshaping the narrative about the so-called rural demise and reframing the story about the place she calls home.

Rural communities are not a monolith of white, impoverished people or a single culture. They represent a diversity of experiences and have been shaped by a diversity of forces. There is no single rural story. That's a significant myth that I am always looking to push back on. —Whitney Kimball Coe

Coe was born and raised in Athens, a small town of about 13,000 between Knoxville and Chattanooga. She was a high school student when she first internalized the message that if you were born in a small town, "success meant getting out," and she fully expected to do just that. But during her undergraduate college years in Charlotte, N.C., Coe had a complete change of heart. "I really missed my home. I felt like I needed Athens, and I discovered that Athens needed me."

After completing an undergraduate degree in religion and philosophy followed by a master's degree in Appalachian studies, Coe moved back home and began working with the Center for Rural Strategies, based out of Whitesburg, Ky. She and her husband are now raising their family in Athens, participating once more in every phase of the small-town life that Coe embraced while growing up. "I'm what people call 'a homecomer,'" she said.

Understanding Population Loss in Rural America

Despite the richness of rural life that is too often overlooked, the data are sobering. For over a century, America's rural population has steadily declined, from a high of 54 percent of the total population in 1910 to just above 19 percent in 2010, according to the latest U.S. Census report.[6] In the past eight years, the number of people living in rural America has continued to drop, from 50 million in 2010 to just above 46 million in 2018.

The population decline can be traced to the consolidation of agriculture and the demise of the family farm, the loss of natural resource and manufacturing jobs, and the exodus of youth, said Mil Duncan, PhD, Professor Emerita of Sociology and founding director of the Carsey Institute at the University of New Hampshire. Although young people have always left rural America, Duncan said that the exodus began to accelerate during the Reagan administration as goods-producing jobs started to disappear and government support for education and economic opportunities simultaneously began to dwindle, a trend that has continued for decades.

Recent reports and headlines highlight many other factors impacting the loss of the rural population. An RWJF-supported *County Health Rankings & Roadmaps* report notes that nearly one in five rural counties has experienced worsening premature death rates over the past decade.[7] The report also noted that no single factor explains this; tobacco and alcohol consumption, lack of access to quality health care, poor housing, food, and limited educational options are all significant contributors.

Clearly, the surge in opioid use in rural areas and the epidemic's death rates have had a devastating impact. (For a comprehensive look at this country's opioid epidemic and its disproportionate impact on rural communities, see Chapter 7, "The Opioid Epidemic: Busting Myths and Sharing Solutions.") A majority of rural Americans view opioid addiction as a problem in their local community, and almost half say it's grown worse in the past five years, according to "Life in Rural America," a 2018 survey report developed by National Public Radio, the Robert Wood Johnson Foundation, and the Harvard T. H. Chan School of Public Health. What's more, the survey found that about three in ten rural Americans say suicide is a serious problem, and more than one in ten say it is a very serious problem.[8]

As rural populations age and die and younger generations leave, Duncan recalled how Carsey demographer Ken Johnson described the changing landscape and population decline: "Coffins outnumber the cradles." And as the economy shifts away from goods-producing jobs, Duncan noted, "we also are seeing lower labor force participation and increasing reliance on disability payments in rural America."

According to a 2018 *New York Times* analysis, economic growth today simply bypasses most rural areas; counties with fewer than 100,000 people lost 17,500 businesses in the first four years of the recovery after the 2008 recession, even as businesses in larger counties expanded.[9]

"The rural economy is struggling, but it still has significant growth potential," said Mark Drabenstott, chairman of MarketSquare, Inc. and the former director of the Federal Reserve's Center for the Study of Rural America. "The question is: 'What is the economic prescription?'"

Fortunately, there are some very promising answers to that question. Drabenstott suggests that unlocking the rural economy's potential will require leaders to collaborate "across state and county lines, and cultivate home-grown businesses instead of chasing smokestacks." *County Health Rankings & Roadmaps* reinforces the idea that access to education, employment, social support, quality housing, and a safe physical environment helps build healthier rural communities.[10]

A body of research documenting the power of education to transform lives is especially compelling. (This topic is explored in greater depth in Chapter 4, "Linking Education and Health to Support the Whole Child.") For example, a report by the Virginia Commonwealth University Center on Society and Health, produced through an RWJF grant, found that Americans with more education live longer, healthier lives than those with fewer years of schooling.[11]

But the consequences of inadequate investments in education are also well documented. Create a map showing where 20 percent of rural America is chronically poor, "and overlay that map with the proportion of people who lack high school educations; it's virtually identical," said the University of New Hampshire's Mil Duncan. "The lack of education leads to vulnerability. When we allow poor education and poor schools to persist, we're trapping these rural people and places in poverty."

Some pathways to change may be more challenging than others. Duncan says research shows that where you live matters when it comes to poverty's impact, an observation that echoes research conducted by Stanford University's Raj Chetty. In separate studies from the 1990s and 2013, Duncan saw that poverty impacts rural communities differently, depending on a region's historical civic and social structures. For example, she found that in rural Appalachia and in the Mississippi Delta a relatively weak and divided system of social and civic institutions led to the vulnerability and exclusion of the poor in everything from jobs to education. By contrast, in poor, rural New England mill towns, she found that strong institutions, a tradition of class integration, and a solid civic culture resulted in a "stable if not vibrant economic path forward."

Unlocking the resources that could make rural communities flourish begins with recognizing that "rural matters." Coe explains why: "Rural matters to the future of our country, in part because nearly 50 million of us live and work in rural areas. We matter as stewards of our nation's natural resources, producers of food, and as the source of large numbers of volunteers for the military. We are part of the equation for achieving a greener, cleaner, and more inclusive country."

Rural futures and urban futures are so interconnected, and we are dependent on one another. —Whitney Kimball Coe

Finding Solutions in the Mid South

Every morning, Ivye L. Allen wakes up to a daunting fact: She is trying to improve the lives of people in three states where the poverty rate is more than 40 percent higher than the national average. That's because the combined poverty rate in Arkansas, Louisiana, and Mississippi—the three states that Allen serves in her role as president of the Foundation for the Mid South—is 18.4 percent, compared to a national poverty rate of 12.8 percent, according to U.S. Census Bureau statistics from 2015 to 2017.[12]

Established in 1990 in Jackson, Miss., the Foundation for the Mid South brings together the public and private sectors and helps them focus their grant resources on increasing long-term social and economic opportunities in the region. In the last two decades, the foundation has secured grants valued at over $750 million to help community organizations create solutions in four key areas that Allen calls "the bedrock" for improved lives and prosperous communities: education, health and wellness, financial security and asset building, and community development.

"What makes us unique is that unlike many community foundations, we serve three states entirely with a goal to have improved outcomes for children and families within the region," said Allen. "Our activities are interrelated, straightforward, and long-term. And at the end of the day, all contribute to healthy communities and improved family outcomes."

Leveraging Resources and People for the Long Term

When Allen first joined the foundation in 2007, she recognized that its grant programs weren't necessarily creating sustainable solutions. So Allen adopted a different approach to help communities move out of poverty by asking, "How do we help people leverage what they have and see what their own strengths are? How do we get people to make an investment in what they have? How do we get the employees and other folks to come to the table and use their resources for what works for the community?" The answer? "By working in strategic partnerships to make public- and private-sector dollars work smarter and increase social and economic opportunities."

As an example of making dollars "work smarter," Allen recalled a Mid South Foundation program that successfully trained nurses for two rural hospitals, each with 100-person staffs. Because hospitals often are considered anchor institutions for their communities—providing jobs, health care, and essential tax revenues—keeping them open and adequately staffed is critical. Allen soon realized, however, that larger medical facilities in Jackson, Miss., and Memphis,

Tenn., were recruiting the new nurses and "plucking them out" of the rural community hospitals.

"So we asked, 'How do we revisit that training and think about it differently?' Now we're looking at and training people who are a little bit more bound to home, getting them the education and skills to be able to provide for their family but they're more likely to stay. And we're very proud of that."

New Language Around the Table

Allen introduced new language to describe the Mid South Foundation's mission: *comprehensive community change.* To better understand the landscape behind this mission, she routinely drives the long stretches of back roads that connect disparate rural communities in order to sit at the table with local people. Allen discourages anyone from "one-and-done" grant perspectives; she helps the stakeholders and local politicians seated beside her see that grant money has to build on existing resources and be locally sustainable if their rural communities are going to survive.

"We work a lot with state government, but I always tell people that we don't necessarily get the resources or policies through the legislature," said Allen. "We get them through practice and long-term relationships with people who are in local positions and jobs, regardless of who's the governor. We really try to be intentional about doing it that way in order to leverage local resources, but also to leverage some changes in behaviors and attitudes. One of the things we do try to be intentional about is strengthening the capacities and knowledge of folks locally to be able to be the champions."

> We don't just invest to invest. We really try to take a partnership approach to the work that we do in order to see bright spots. —Ivye L. Allen

Along with business, the foundation partners with local government agencies and community development organizations, such as the Mississippi Delta Workforce Funding Collaborative, to provide workforce education, training, and small business development opportunities. This type of partnership came into play recently in Cleveland, Miss., one of the poorest rural areas in the country. The depths of the area's poverty are long-standing, first drawing the world's attention back in 1967, when Senator Robert F. Kennedy toured the Mississippi Delta. After visiting an impoverished Cleveland neighborhood where 15 people lived in a dilapidated, unheated shack with only a jar of peanut butter for food, Kennedy reportedly said, "I've been to third-world countries and I've never seen anything like this."[13]

Recently, after several big chain pharmacies opened their doors, a nonprofit group alerted Allen that pharmacy technicians were needed in the area. Allen started networking, finding partners who could help identify and train potential pharmacy tech candidates. Soon, a community college instructor in Cleveland agreed to teach classes at night, and a $50,000 grant paved the way for 20 local citizens to attend the program and become pharmacy technicians at Walgreens, CVS, and the local hospital.

Allen will never forget that graduation ceremony: "I could tell that some of those individuals had to borrow the clothes that they were wearing for their graduation. But at the end of the day, they had their kids there to watch them succeed in something. And it said to them that they could take care of their families. That's $50,000 well spent."

Looking Behind the Numbers

The Foundation for the Mid South purposefully works with employers looking to hire 10 to 20 people. That's not a headline-grabbing scale, but to Allen it's all about perspective—and the importance of looking behind those numbers.

"When we talk numbers only, we lose some great stories," she said. "We can't just look at the one individual doing the job training or the one individual completing that GED, because oftentimes there's a family behind an adult doing it. And if there are 10 people we helped to work, those 10 people really probably impacted 45. In these communities, that really counts."

Many of the programs supported by the foundation are specifically designed to enhance access to economic mobility in a rural setting. For example, the foundation has supported:

- Rental car programs that help people without cars get to work; purchase of tools needed to take a new job; and child care facilities, in partnership with nonprofits and churches.
- Creation of the Mississippi Reentry Guide, a collaboration with local leaders and the Mississippi Reentry Council, to connect ex-offenders with services and agencies that support successful transitions back to their communities.
- Strategies to improve high school graduation rates, workforce preparedness, and life outcomes, in partnership with nonprofit organizations. One such approach is the Males of Color initiative, which focuses on tutoring, mentoring, career development, and life-learning strategies for young men at risk of not finishing high school.
- Development of green spaces, community parks, hospitals, and grocery stores that enhance healthier lifestyles.

A Native Daughter Who Found Her Voice

As everyone around her can appreciate, Allen honestly talks the talk when it comes to the Mid South region. A native of Greeneville, Miss., she moved to New York City after graduating from Howard University to pursue degrees from Hunter College, New York University, and a PhD in social policy from Columbia University. She then worked in finance and marketing for Fortune 100 corporations and directed fellowship programs for the Rockefeller Brothers Fund.

When her mother asked, Allen said repeatedly that she "didn't see herself coming back" to her Southern roots. But as her work with philanthropy expanded, "I remembered my own upbringing and how much talent was there. The opportunity came, and I ended up being able to come back close to home."

Like Coe, Allen is now a homecomer, and 13 years later she has never regretted her decision. "When I look at the people here, I see lots of hope. I see people with dreams. It's an ongoing journey, but overall we can see the fruit of our investment, our engagement. Is it always to the magnitude or the level we envision? No. But being able to see the needle move is great."

Hope for the Town "Where the Southern Crosses the Yellow Dog"

Moorhead, Miss., is a quiet town, defined by two railroad tracks (one still used, one defunct), scattered one-story homes, and a smattering of small-town amenities in the shadows of long-gone textile mills. There is a Dollar General, an auto parts store, a few churches, a gas station, the post office, a convenience store, two local schools, and a branch of Mississippi Delta Community College. The welcome sign at the edge of town reminds visitors that Moorhead was the hometown of Grand Old Opry star John Russell, which explains Johnny Russell Drive in front of the public library.

There is also a historical Mississippi Blues Trail marker in the shadows of the town's water tower explaining Moorhead's claim to fame as the spot "where the Southern crosses the Yellow Dog." It reads:

> *The junction of the Southern Railroad and the Yazoo Delta Railroad (the "Yellow Dog") was established in 1897. For decades it was the central Delta's major rail link, making Moorhead one of the region's most active passenger and freight connections. The crossing gained national fame in 1914 with W. C. Handy's seminal blues song, "The Yellow Dog Rag."*

When HOPE leaders visited Moorhead in 2014, one thing was clear: Whatever was left of Moorhead's once thriving community fabric was hanging on by a thread. This struggling enclave of 2,200 people, 88 percent black and 49 percent poor, had a single bank, a Regions Bank branch. But the institution offered limited services and had recently made the business decision to exit the market. A number of residents relied on the lone gas station inside the town limits to conduct financial transactions.

"Throughout the Delta, it's not uncommon for residents to bank at the town gas station," said Ed Sivak, executive vice president for policy and communications for HOPE. "Residents will frequently turn to the gas stations to purchase money orders, sometimes several at one time, to pay bills."

The Unbanked Get a Financial Home

Regions Bank officials asked HOPE if it would consider taking over the branch to ensure that banking services remained available in the community. With locations in five Deep South states, HOPE works predominantly in economically distressed rural communities, many in persistent poverty counties with a poverty rate that has exceeded 20 percent for three decades.

Founded in 1994, HOPE, a community development financial institution, credit union, and policy institute, has generated some $2.5 billion in financing. Collectively, projects supported by HOPE and its advocacy have benefited more than one million individuals in Alabama, Arkansas, Louisiana, Mississippi, and Tennessee.[14] HOPE advances the goal of financial inclusion by banking the unbanked, expanding access to capital for disadvantaged businesses, making mortgage loans to first-time homeowners, and investing in high-impact community resources such as rural hospitals, schools, grocery stores, and affordable housing. Through these strategies, HOPE, a minority- and women-owned financial institution, builds wealth among historically underserved populations.

Sivak anchors all conversations about HOPE in his belief that economic mobility and access to financial services are inextricably connected. Simply stated, Sivak believes that the ability to improve lives in rural America and create pathways out of persistent poverty are directly linked to a person's access to a job and a bank account.

The most important relationship one will have with the economy is his or her job. And the second most important relationship is the one that he or she will have with a financial institution. —Ed Sivak

When economic mobility is low, he explained, "organizations and social services focus on basic needs. But as mobility increases, residents gain access to institutions that provide living wages and facilitate asset accumulation. They have access to more opportunities."

Sivak cites compelling statistics about the wealth gap to highlight the importance of access to capital: on average, white Americans as a whole have a median net worth 13 times the net worth of black Americans;[15] however, the net worth of white business owners shrinks to three times that of black business owners. That, he said, clearly supports the argument that expanding access to capital—particularly among people of color—is a viable strategy to close the wealth gap attributable to race.

In 2015, with the support from Regions Bank, HOPE opened a credit union in the former Regions Bank building, catty-corner from that Yellow Dog historical marker. Credit union members can now open checking accounts, apply for loans, and take out cash from the town's first bank ATM, which HOPE installed in the branch.

"When we opened," Sivak remembers, "we literally had people walk two miles to the credit union branch to borrow money to get the resources they needed. And we aren't talking about money for vacations or new dining room furniture. One person needed to repair a truck that had been sitting idle for months, another had to have help to buy a car. In a rural community, you have to have a car or you don't have access to employment, a doctor, a grocery store. You have to have mobility."

From Transactions to Transformations

Over time, HOPE has supported a wide range of Moorhead community projects: a new walking trail and renovated baseball fields at the city park, along with improved restrooms; training for community leaders through a NeighborWorks Community Leadership Institute; and plans to create more affordable housing, a top priority for the town. "Almost everything we do is in some way connected to improving some aspect with the social determinants of health," Sivak said.

He has always insisted that when HOPE enters a community, "We are not just about transactions. We ask, 'How can we be involved in transformation?'" Toward that goal, HOPE initiated the Small Towns Partnership program, which provides strategic and focused community and economic development training and technical assistance where none had previously existed.

The ultimate goals of the partnership are to advance key community development projects, attract private and public resources, expand economic opportunity, and build the financial capability of the communities and their residents. "Development solutions rest with local people," Sivak said, echoing a core belief of the Mid South Foundation's Ivye Allen, who serves on HOPE's board of directors. "The only pathways to sustainability are going to be the solutions that have the full involvement and investment of local people."

HOPE's effort to prioritize development strategies grounded in the will of local people was evident in its work with a tattered housing subdivision called Eastmoor, just outside Moorhead's town limits. "It was literally built to disenfranchise black voters, to move just enough black residents out of town to maintain a white majority to elect a white mayor," said Sivak. Indeed, the place had become a virtual killing field. Of the 60 or so original homes, approximately 20 had burned to the ground because of shoddy wiring and poor gas connections. A local resident had died of a heart attack after spending hours digging a trench to redirect the sewage that had filled his front yard.

Shortly after Bill Bynum, HOPE's chief executive officer, arrived in Moorhead, Mayor George Holland directed him to Eastmoor for a tour. According to Sivak, Bynum turned first to Eastmoor's local leaders. Seated one day in the home of the community association president, in a kitchen with a collapsed ceiling and exposed roof rafters, Bynum asked, "What does the community need?" And she replied, "All I want for this community is streets without cracks so the elderly folks can go visit their neighbors without having to trip. And a new playground for the children."

Recounting Bynum's visit to Eastmoor, Sivak said he was stunned by that answer. "She didn't say, 'A new home, or a new roof, or a new ceiling.' She talked about her community, not herself. Today, we're rebuilding every home in this community, and a playground. This is 'home' from the front end."

The Impact of HOPE

HOPE's impact can be seen in any number of projects throughout the Deep South:

- In Gloster, Miss., HOPE helped finance a new local grocery store for residents who previously had to drive nearly an hour to buy fresh food at an affordable price. "We haven't felt like human beings here for years, and now we do," one shopper told the owner of the new store.
- In Drew, Miss., HOPE is exploring options to turn an empty school building in the middle of town into affordable housing. The building has historical significance: It was built by Julius Rosenwald, former president of Sears, who

once teamed up with noted American educator Booker T. Washington to build schools across the South for black children.

- In Ferriday, La., HOPE helped secure financing for a rural hospital that will modernize the delivery of health care and serve as an anchor institution in the local economy.
- In Birmingham, Ala., HOPE provided $9 million in New Market Tax Credits to finance a new building project for the A. G. Gaston Boys & Girls Club, HOPE's first major investment in Alabama. The project will increase the organization's capacity to offer tutoring and mentoring services to youth.
- In Little Rock, Ark., HOPE opened a credit union branch in a predominantly Hispanic community to expand access to financial services for Latino immigrants.

As it celebrates its 25th anniversary, HOPE is recognized as one of the nation's leading CDFIs in underserved communities. In 2018, HOPE won the *Wall Street Journal* Financial Inclusion Challenge, in part for opening a cluster of credit union branches in the Mississippi Delta. On February 18, 2019, NBC's *Today* show featured HOPE's work to close financial service gaps in the Deep South. And in June 2019, HOPE was one of two organizations recognized nationally by the National Housing Conference for its work to advance affordable housing.

Sivak knows the effort to achieve economic inclusion is never ending, particularly in light of glaring resource inequities. The issue of persistent poverty in this country is "largely a rural phenomenon," he explained, but the funding available for community development "can skew urban. That's a resource concern."

Sivak doesn't just call out public dollars in that analysis, he includes philanthropic giving as well. According to "As the South Grows," a report by the National Committee for Responsive Philanthropy and Grantmakers for Southern Progress, per capita grantmaking in the Alabama Black Belt and the Mississippi Delta regions is about "$41 per person between 2010 and 2014, compared to a national funding rate of $451 per person and the New York City rate of $1,996 per person."[16]

> *Our work provides an opportunity to address the structures that have created these inequalities in the first place. The presence or absence of a financial institution that meets people where they are is going to signal how wide or narrow a mobility path will be within any community. —Ed Sivak*

Center for Rural Strategies

The Center for Rural Strategies, where Whitney Kimball Coe serves as national program director, seeks to improve economic and social conditions through the creative and innovative use of media and communications. By presenting accurate and compelling portraits of rural lives and cultures, Rural Strategies hopes to deepen public debate and create an environment in which positive change for rural communities in the United States and around the world can occur. (The media's power to help frame that kind of issue and raise its visibility on the national agenda is described in Chapter 2, "How Media Shape the Public Discourse and Influence Health.")

As it delivers fresh insights about rural conditions, the center also strives to create better economic and social opportunities through coalition building, partnerships, and public information campaigns, while advancing strategies that strengthen the connections between rural and urban places.[17] Among its key projects:

- The *Daily Yonder*, an online platform that covers rural news for a national audience, including rural residents, advocates, policymakers, and journalists. In addition to Coe's recent column in response to the *New York Times,* topics have included the impact of the government shutdown on rural communities, efforts by hog farmers in North Carolina to deal with hog lagoon waste, the impact of telehealth on rural communities, investment in rural communities as the next big opportunity, Navajo LGBTQ youth and their elder champions, the geography of food support programs, and the pharmaceutical companies behind the opioid epidemic.
- The *Rural Assembly*, a rural movement of organizations and individuals from all 50 states working at local, regional, and national levels to usher in a more inclusive nation that values all people, no matter their zip code. Established in 2007 and coordinated by Coe, the Rural Assembly has become a strong and effective advocate for rural places, people, and issues. Its participants represent the diversity of rural cultures, races, and geographies, and include local grassroots organizers, nonprofit and business leaders, government officials, funders, and next-generation leaders. In December 2018, the Center for Rural Strategies received a two-year grant from RWJF to support the work of the Rural Assembly.[18]
- The *Rural Broadband Policy Group*, a national coalition of rural and urban groups working together to create better broadband access for rural America and other marginalized communities. Over 30 percent of rural Americans do not have access to broadband at home, compared to 4 percent of urban Americans—a digital, discriminatory divide that impacts how rural Americans

can participate in the economy, enjoy modern conveniences, and access educational and health care resources across all age groups. A 2018 policy report, supported by the Center for Rural Strategies and ThinkTennessee, a nonpartisan think tank, noted that Tennessee is ranked 44th in the nation for broadband subscribers, and offered solutions to help bridge the digital gap.[19]

Coe believes that every national issue plays out on a rural scale—including migrant labor, immigration, the opioid epidemic, climate change, and health care—and rural places often address them in ways that challenge traditional narratives. Describing a recent U.S. Immigration and Customs Enforcement (ICE) raid at a meatpacking plant in Morristown, Tenn., a small rural area north of Athens, she was struck by how the community came together. "The community schools, churches, and businesses just rose up and supported all of these families who had lost loved ones to this raid and were going to be deported, creating space for these families to feel safe and supported."

A local Baptist pastor spoke out clearly about it, she recalled.[20] "He said, 'These people are part of our community.' And I think that gets to the heart of the rural essence, our lived experience: staying in relationships with the people right in front of you."

Coe's views on rural America, and the work of the Center for Rural Strategies, have emerged as assertive voices of rural engagement. Over the last two years, she has spoken at RWJF's *Sharing Knowledge* conference, been a guest on the National Public Radio program, *On Being with Krista Tippett,* and worn her Dolly Parton T-shirt and denim jacket to discuss "Rural by Choice" at the Aspen Ideas Festival.

And at the inaugural Obama Foundation Summit in Chicago in October 2017, in a moving speech called "Practicing the Small-Town Art of Participation," Coe spoke of the challenges and rich rewards that come with living in rural America:

> *"We keep showing up. At funerals and potlucks. At PTA meetings and choir practice. At football games and city council meetings. We keep checking out library books and performing in community theater productions. And that regular practice of participation is what characterizes our relationships, and that gives us the ability to live and work and worship together in spite of disagreements. . . .*
>
> *"I believe there is something incredibly powerful about the way we show up with each other in small, daily ways. The way we stay within sight and sound of each other. It's a practice. That's the only word I can think of to describe what we do. . . . On the one hand, we are not doing anything new or brilliant. We are just modeling the practices that we grew up on. But I do believe that we are doing the thing that is truly necessary right now, in this time*

of divisiveness and polarization across every kind of border. We are doing the hard work of staying in community."

The audience rose as one when Coe finished her speech, giving her a standing ovation.

A Final Word

RWJF is committed to supporting the efforts of rural communities and their residents to live the healthiest lives possible. In addition to supporting research and emerging insights into the many sides of rural health in America, the Foundation helps support and lift up community-driven solutions and initiatives that leverage local resources and strengths, such as strong social connections and civic engagement, that have been linked to good health.

These RWJF efforts include programs that bridge gaps in health care for rural and underserved communities; promote physical, emotional, and cultural well-being; improve social and economic opportunities for people living in rural America; and foster a sense of belonging and a shared vision of health for all. For instance, one initiative called *Project ECHO* uses ongoing telementoring to equip primary care practitioners in rural areas with the knowledge they need to provide high-quality specialty care, while another initiative called *Well-Connected Communities* equips volunteer leaders to help their neighbors be healthier at every stage of life. These efforts provide pathways to change that ideally allow rural communities to move away from poverty without losing their unique rural identities and strengths.

At RWJF's "Life in Rural America Symposium," held May 2019 in Charleston, W.Va., rural and tribal experts from across the country discussed strategies to propel health equity in rural America, and heard the results of the two-part "Life in Rural America" survey.[21] Despite the most recent findings that four in ten rural Americans face challenges to good health that include financial insecurity and trouble accessing affordable health care and housing, rural Americans also continue to be optimistic and satisfied with their quality of life and feel safe in their communities.

"We believe the results of these surveys are unique in their focus on individuals' personal experiences in their rural communities across a range of areas of life," said Carolyn Miller, RWJF senior program officer who helped coordinate the May 2019 symposium. "The findings will provide us with important evidence on how realities look on the ground across rural America, and give us an opportunity to start a grounded conversation about health, well-being, and equity in rural America."

Linking Education and Health to Support the Whole Child

Sarah M. Lee, PhD, Team Lead, School Health Branch, Division of Population Health, Centers for Disease Control and Prevention

Jason Q. Purnell, PhD, Associate Professor, Brown School, Washington University in St. Louis

Loel Solomon, PhD, Vice President, Community Health, Kaiser Permanente

(The findings and conclusions in this chapter are those of the authors and do not necessarily represent the official position of the Centers for Disease Control and Prevention.)

Young people, from toddlers in preschool to teens in high school, spend most of their nonfamily time in an educational setting, an experience that is critical to their developmental, health, and life outcomes. Children and youth who are supported in being physically active, eating healthy diets, refraining from substance use, and developing other healthy habits perform better in school, and better educated people are healthier and live longer.[1]

The complex, bidirectional connection between education and health can foster opportunity, making it a key component of the mantra, "Health starts where we live, learn, work, and play."

Yet access to quality education and the knowledge and foundation it provides are not distributed equitably. Schools located in areas of concentrated poverty often lack resources to fully provide even the basic academic materials and supports needed for an adequate educational experience, let alone the complete range of associated services that can help ensure a child's educational and developmental success. By making the commitments needed to support the whole child, schools, families, health care providers, and communities can help ensure that children across all population groups and geographic regions can succeed.

Culture of Health in Practice, Alonzo L. Plough. Oxford University Press (2020) © Robert Wood Johnson Foundation
DOI: 10.1093/oso/9780190071400.001.0001

The contributors to this chapter present a compelling case for school health models designed to maximize every child's prospects for the learning and personal health achievements that are the ingredients of a satisfying life. Sarah Lee reviews the factors that can influence educational success and explains the evolution of the Whole School, Whole Community, Whole Child (WSCC) model, which is a comprehensive way to connect education and health. Jason Purnell describes an initiative designed to expand implementation of WSCC across the United States, with a focus on under-resourced school districts, while Loel Solomon details Kaiser Permanente's work to support student and school staff health and resilience, which also builds on a commitment to the whole child framework.

An Inequitable Landscape

A healthy body, mind, and spirit—the prerequisites for realizing educational potential—are elusive goals for many children whose childhoods are spent in environments that lack the resources needed to support their healthy development and learning. Multiple studies have found that educational outcomes can vary by race, ethnicity, socioeconomic status, and geographic location; by the adversity faced by children who grow up in difficult circumstances; and by unhealthy behaviors that result from lack of knowledge and opportunity.

Sarah Lee, at the Centers for Disease Control and Prevention (CDC), pointed to a range of data that illustrate some of the inequities.

Baseline: High School Graduation and Success in Math and Reading

Key differences in the fundamental measures of high school graduation and mastery of high school-level math and reading are evident by race, ethnicity, and geography:

- Approximately 12 percent of adults ages 25 and older do not have a high school diploma. The highest concentrations of adults without that degree are in areas with poorer health outcomes, especially the Southeast, the Southwest, and certain regions of California.[2]
- Eighty-four percent of students in U.S. public high schools graduated within four years of starting ninth grade, according to the most recent data available (2014–2015 school year). But disparities by racial and ethnic group are dramatic, with the graduation rate for American Indians/Alaska Natives

at 72 percent and just slightly higher for non-Hispanic blacks (76%) and Hispanics (79%). By comparison, 88 percent of non-Hispanic whites and 91 percent of Asians/Pacific Islanders graduate within four years.[3]

- Asian 12th-grade students scored 11 points higher in math in the 2015 National Assessment of Educational Progress (NAEP), on average, compared with scores for non-Hispanic white students in the same grade. Other racial and ethnic groups scored comparatively worse: Hispanic students scored 32 points lower, American Indian/Alaska Native students 33 points lower, and non-Hispanic black students 41 points lower, compared with Asian students.[4]
- Average 12th-grade 2015 NAEP reading scores for Asian students were two points above those of non-Hispanic white students; the scores of American Indian/Alaska Native students were 18 points lower, Hispanic students 21 points lower, and non-Hispanic black students 31 points lower than Asian students.[5]

Growing Up at a Disadvantage and Suffering the Consequences

Family and community issues—including poverty, poor nutrition, violence, un-addressed chronic health conditions, and the disruptions associated with un-employment and incarceration—can impact both a child's health and readiness to learn.

Lee sketched the breadth of the problem by presenting government data from many sources that tracked potential learning barriers for students in various age groups. Their home environments were major contributors, given the finding that 21 percent of students live in poverty,[6] 31 percent in a single-parent household,[7] and 8 percent in a food-insecure household.[8] Other significant hurdles included mental and behavioral health issues, such as experiencing a mental disorder (up to 20% of students[9,10,11]), being bullied (19% of high school students[12]), and suffering abuse each year (674,000 children under age 18 in 2017[13]). Not getting enough sleep is another impediment to learning for the majority (75%) of students.[14]

People who suffered adverse childhood experiences (ACEs), such as those mentioned above, are at increased risk for many negative health outcomes (such as cancer, diabetes, heart disease, and mental health disorders) and behaviors (including alcohol and drug use, physical inactivity, smoking, and unsafe sexual practices).

The impact of ACEs increases with the number of adverse experiences and extends to other dimensions of well-being. Compared with people who have not faced any ACEs, those who have experienced four or more double their risk of not completing high school and are at nearly two-and-a-half times the risk of being unemployed. They are also 50 percent more likely to live in poverty. A cross-generational impact is evident as well, with research indicating that lower parental education, employment, and income increase the risk of poor educational outcomes for their children, from age 4 and throughout their schooling.[15]

Differences in the experience of ACEs are evident by race and ethnicity, with prevalence highest among non-Hispanic black children and lowest among Asian children: 61 percent and 23 percent, respectively, have encountered at least one ACE. Some 51 percent of Hispanic children and 40 percent of non-Hispanic white children have had at least one ACE.[16]

The Impact of Behavior

Strong evidence from a range of sources supports the links between healthy eating and academic achievement and between physical activity and academic achievement.[17,18] Students who participate in the U.S. Department of Agriculture (USDA) School Breakfast Program tend to earn higher grades, perform better on standardized tests, are less likely to be absent from school, and have better memories. Likewise, physically active students tend to have higher grades and a better record in terms of school attendance and classroom behavior. Data also show that recess time improves cognitive performance (as reflected in factors such as attention) and classroom behavior.

By contrast, researchers have found an association between lower grades and both student hunger and inadequate consumption of fruits, vegetables, or dairy products. Students who are hungry are also more likely to be absent from school and to have difficulty focusing.

Student self-reports also demonstrate a connection between healthy behavior and academic outcomes. The CDC's 2015 Youth Risk Behavior Survey of students from ninth to twelfth grades identified these links:[19]

- Students report higher grades (A's and B's) if they are physically active at least 60 minutes on five or more days each week or play at least one team sport. They are more likely to have lower grades (C's and D's) if they watch television, play video or computer games, or use a computer for other than school work for three or more hours daily.
- Higher grades are associated with several dietary patterns: eating breakfast every day, eating fruits and vegetables every day, drinking milk every day, and not drinking soda.
- Lower grades are associated with using marijuana, cocaine, heroin, and methamphetamines and with attempting suicide. Lower grades are also associated with staying out of school due to concerns about safety.

Yet, despite all that we know about the influence of nutrition, physical activity, substance use, and other behaviors on educational outcomes, engagement in healthy behaviors varies greatly across population groups. The 2017 Youth Risk Behavior Survey generated a vast dataset on behaviors that promote or undermine health.[20] A few examples:

- Compared with other racial and ethnic groups, non-Hispanic black and Hispanic students are less likely to be physically active at least 60 minutes on five or more days weekly and more likely to watch television three or more hours per day.
- Non-Hispanic white students are more likely than Hispanic and non-Hispanic black students to have tried cigarette smoking and to be current smokers.
- Non-Hispanic black students are less likely than Hispanic or non-Hispanic white students to consume fruits and vegetables or to eat breakfast every day.
- Non-Hispanic white students are more likely to use alcohol currently than Hispanics and much more likely than non-Hispanic black students.
- Both non-Hispanic black and Hispanic students are more likely to skip school due to concerns about safety.

Clearly, underlying social and economic conditions influence the health-related behaviors of young people and, in turn, their educational outcomes. Given the scope of the responsibility that is lodged in the schools, and the limits of their resources, especially in disadvantaged communities, the challenge of mitigating harms and promoting practices that can lift up health and achievement in educational settings remains enormous.

"We're missing the mark in educating the most vulnerable young people," said Jason Purnell of Washington University in St. Louis. "We have to start asking some fundamental questions connected to health first and retool education—for all children, but particularly for the most vulnerable."

Right now, the focus is on drilling children with academic skills who maybe haven't eaten or who have been traumatized, and then wondering why that's not working. —Jason Purnell

A School Health Model for the Whole Child

The CDC has funded school health for 25 years, helping to evolve an integrated model designed to address children's needs holistically by considering the factors that influence the education–health connection, including poverty and family and community dynamics and support. This emphasis on the "whole child" has gained traction within the education field during this period and underlies current thinking about how best to promote student academic achievement, health, and well-being.

An Integrated and Comprehensive Approach

In the early 1990s, the CDC's Division of Adolescent and School Health adopted the Coordinated School Health Model,[21] which Lee described as a "systematic, synergistic approach." It included eight components: healthy school environment; health education; health services; nutrition services; counseling, psychological, and social services; physical education; health promotion for staff; and family/community involvement.

Separately, the education-focused organization ASCD (formerly Association for Supervision and Curriculum Development) launched its Whole Child approach in 2007, directed primarily at the education sector, including its leaders.[22] This represented a shift from a narrower academic definition of achievement to a vision that supported children's long-term development and success.

The existence of two models, and the unclear connection between them, caused some confusion in the field, leading the CDC and ASCD to collaborate on refining and combining their approaches. Their partnership led to the development and launch in 2014 of the powerful Whole School, Whole Community, Whole Child (WSCC) model.[23, 24] "That re-ignited an emphasis and interest in school health," said Lee. She added that the strength of WSCC lies in the evidence-based strategies for implementing each component of the model.

WSCC's framework places the student at its center, surrounded by the interconnected factors that support good health and educational outcomes. The core principle underlying the model, said Purnell, is that "children are sustained in feeling healthy, safe, engaged, supported, and challenged." The 10 components that surround the child are the "aspects of health that need to be not just present in schools and school systems, but, more importantly, integrated and coordinated among a set of school and community partners." These components are:

- Health education
- Physical education and physical activity
- Nutrition environment and services
- Health services
- Counseling, psychological, and social services
- Social and emotional climate
- Physical environment
- Employee wellness
- Family engagement
- Community involvement

"This can't be just another thing we put on the plates of school administrators," Purnell stressed. "Communities must think differently about the ways in which they support schools, including a rational and robust way of partnering with service providers, programs, and other resources that can support children, faculty, and staff within schools." Thus, community forms the model's border.

A special 2015 issue of the *Journal of School Health* explains all aspects of WSCC in detail.[25]

Taking the Model to Scale

In 2014, researchers at Washington University issued "For the Sake of All," a report examining the health and well-being of African Americans in St. Louis. From there, the research team developed a body of work, which became known as Health Equity Works, designed to translate the report's findings into actionable strategies that address health equity. By 2016, one of those strategies involved a focus on the WSCC model.

As the Washington University team began to convene stakeholders in the St. Louis region to consider how to go deeper in its work, they became aware of—and applied for—a new RWJF initiative designed to encourage uptake of the WSCC model across the United States. Out of more than 80 applications, Washington University became one of three partners in *Together for Healthy and Successful Schools*, each with its own role in the initiative:

- *Washington University*, through Health Equity Works at the Brown School: Developing a research-based, user-friendly toolkit for school leaders.
- *America's Promise Alliance*: Learning how to support health and well-being in schools at six sites across the country, tapping into its networks, and bringing in youth voices to make the case for healthy schools.
- *Child Trends*: Creating policy tools and research-based model policies for educators, policymakers, and the public.

"One of the chief strengths of WSCC," said Purnell, "is its comprehensiveness, which is also a challenge. It is so comprehensive that it can become overwhelming, particularly for schools and districts that serve the most vulnerable populations." The Washington University researchers are intentionally exploring how WSCC can work in school districts that serve high-need student populations. The logic, said Purnell, is, "If you can make it work in a district with perhaps fewer resources and higher needs, then you can make it work in districts where there are more resources."

The main research question for the Washington University research team is: What are the conditions necessary to move from the WSCC framework to its implementation? "Frameworks don't implement themselves," Purnell observed. "Human beings, embedded in systems and armed with messages, implement frameworks. We don't often give enough thought to the human dynamics at play when trying to implement models like WSCC."

To uncover those dynamics, research partners from the Brown School and from the Center on Society and Health at Virginia Commonwealth University are thinking creatively about the broader adoption of WSCC, using social network analysis, communications science, system dynamics, implementation science, and other methodologies. A national advisory committee with representatives from across the education–health spectrum is offering guidance on how best to disseminate this work in the hopes of making WSCC nationally viable.

Designing the Blueprint in St. Louis

In keeping with an emphasis on the potential to implement WSCC in high-need schools and districts, the Washington University team has focused on the St. Louis Public Schools District, which serves over 20,000 children, and Normandy Schools Collaborative, an inner-ring suburban district just outside St. Louis serving about 6,000 students. Both districts face significant challenges and are open to thinking about new ways to support children.

The research team brings extensive experience with St. Louis schools and a cross-sector working group that focuses on using school-based health centers to improve health and educational outcomes. As of the 2019–2020 school year, six of the ten highest-need high schools in St. Louis will have a school-based health center. What began as a St. Louis–based working group has evolved into a state affiliate of the School-Based Health Alliance with a mission to support school-based health care throughout the state of Missouri.

The research in the St. Louis and the Normandy districts involves a multistep process. Researchers identify the most influential people within a school building or system. "They may not be the usual suspects," said Purnell. "Social network analysis highlights the unusual suspects." Rather than the principal or superintendent, for example, it might be the custodian, the school secretary, or the person who checks students out at the lunch line. Mapping relationships in terms of information flow and trust helps determine the structure of the social network in place, offering guidance about who should be involved in implementation efforts.

Having a more sophisticated sense of the connections between people in the system allows you to target your efforts in a more intelligent way. —Jason Purnell

Researchers are also testing messages: how to talk about the relationship between health and education and about the model "as something that can be a useful tool that helps educators to do their jobs more effectively, rather than the 'reform or model du jour' that they have rightly become skeptical of," said Purnell. Those on the frontlines of education don't need to be convinced that health is important; they do need to understand what to do and how to do it. One of the messages that has most resonated with educators, Purnell said, is that "this isn't the classroom teacher's job alone, or the principal's, or the school nurse's. This is an all-hands-on-deck approach needed to make this part of how schools function."

Finally, the researchers, along with health and education partners, employ systems science to describe the baseline for the district—how health is currently conceptualized, health services are being delivered, and health activities are happening within schools. Then they design an optimal system and figure out what it will take to implement it.

Throughout, and with partners at the Brown School's Social Systems Design Lab, the team uses group model-building techniques in which multiple stakeholders—students, teachers, administrators, parents, community partners—diagram systems within the schools that support health and well-being.

The goal is to develop a toolkit and blueprint for WSCC implementation that accounts for human- and system-level factors and can be used in schools beyond St. Louis and Normandy. It will provide guidance on assessing social networks within a school or district, offering different approaches for schools with varying levels of resources, as well as sample messages to communicate with multiple audiences about WSCC. It will also include a template for bringing diverse stakeholders together for group model building.

> *When implementing anything new, you need to think about the people, the systems, and the messages. —Jason Purnell*

Purnell anticipates different versions of the toolkit. A 1.0 version will likely be web-based with well-designed PDF-format tools, while a 2.0 version may include a more interactive set of resources. These initial sets of tools will be available to all districts at no charge.

The comprehensiveness of the WSCC model moves well beyond the healthy lunches and physical activity frame that many people associate with school health, noted Purnell. Although these are essential elements, the social and emotional well-being of young people has gained attention over time and is well-integrated into the model. Research in St. Louis also has uncovered connections between the health and well-being of the faculty and staff and that of both parents and students. "WSCC provides a framework for thinking about these interlocking components of what makes a healthy school environment and supports the health and well-being of young people," Purnell observed.

Purnell is seeing more interest in WSCC, and his team is actively soliciting that interest through presentations at meetings of school districts across the country. "The word is apparently getting out," he said. "We'd like to make it accessible to districts that may not have a Washington University in their backyard who has gotten a grant from the Robert Wood Johnson Foundation, and help them think through those issues and get to better implementation and hopefully better outcomes."

Child Trends, one of the *Together for Healthy and Successful Schools* partners, has collaborated with the Institute for Health Research and Policy at the University of Illinois at Chicago and EMT Associates Inc. in a study to analyze state educational statutes and regulations to determine how well they are aligned with the WSCC model.[26]

Key findings of the analysis, published in January 2019, include:

- Coverage of the various components of WSCC is "both broad and deep" in 10 states. In 20 states, coverage is "limited or weak," addressing only certain components.
- The WSCC component with least coverage is school-employee wellness, with only Mississippi covering this in a comprehensive way.
- Minimal integration between components is evident, even in states that show broad and deep coverage.

I don't think we're out of the standardized test mania phase, but I think people are open and asking different questions about how we get to better educational outcomes and better developmental outcomes as well for our children. —Jason Purnell

From Shipyards to Classrooms

Kaiser Permanente, the country's largest not-for-profit health plan and a leading integrated health care system, has its roots in the Richmond, Calif., shipyards established by industrialist Henry J. Kaiser, which built cargo ships during World War II. Back then, Kaiser Shipyards opened health care centers to serve its workers—a new form of health care delivery through a prepaid group practice that became the basis of the Kaiser Permanente health plan. When the war ended, the plan was opened to the public, with strong union support.

Child care centers also opened at the Kaiser Shipyards to assist women entering the workforce during the war years. Created by leading child development experts, the centers became a proven model of early childhood education for many years after the war's end. They also offered nutritious meals and an on-site physician and nurse to ensure the health and safety of the workers' children.

"So we had some early experience at the intersection of health and education, with the recognition of how important that was for creating a sense of well-being for workers who were parents," said Kaiser Permanente's Loel Solomon. "We feel that connection today."

Now, one in five Kaiser Permanente members is a school-aged child or a school employee. After reviewing data from more than 60 community interventions implemented over many years, Kaiser Permanente recognized that it could have the largest impact on population health by working in the schools. "It's a captive audience and you are able to implement policy and systems changes with some level of strength," said Solomon.

> We can't be effective in addressing the health and well-being of our members in the communities we serve if we don't go to the settings where people spend most of their day. —Loel Solomon

In 2011, Kaiser Permanente launched Thriving Schools to coordinate and bring focus to its work around school health, with an overarching goal of improving the health of students and staff.[27] With an emphasis on support, safety, engagement, and staff wellness, the Thriving Schools strategy is very much in sync with the whole child model.

Healthy Eating and Active Living

Thriving Schools began with an emphasis on healthy eating and active living (HEAL), bringing the strong evidence base on obesity prevention to a large number of schools.

With 14,000 schools in the eight states plus the District of Columbia where Kaiser Permanente operates, scaling an effective intervention requires strong partnerships. Kaiser Permanente's closest collaborator on HEAL has been the Alliance for a Healthier Generation, which is itself a partnership between the American Heart Association and the Clinton Foundation.

For HEAL, Kaiser Permanente worked with Healthier Generation to introduce Healthier Generation's Healthy Schools Program into 699 Kaiser Permanente–affiliated schools in six regions around the country. Program managers—who work with cohorts of schools and their leadership teams to conduct school assessments, identify opportunities for change, and build leadership—are a key feature of the model, which leverages a powerful evidence base with coaching, technical assistance, action planning, and mentoring. Kaiser Permanente is seeing "exciting changes in food and, in particular, physical activity practices" at the schools in which it is working, said Solomon.

Through HEAL, more exercise has been added to the school day, with an emphasis on physical activity at school beyond gym class, walking and biking to school, and on-campus programs for adults. Headway also has been made on healthy eating, using tactics from behavioral economics to influence consumption patterns in the lunchroom (e.g., putting healthier snacks at the front of a shelf), monitoring food insecurity among students, and increasing participation in free and reduced-cost school lunches. Kaiser Permanente offers mini-grants to schools to encourage the uptake of the most effective strategies.

Labor unions can be allies in integrating wellness into school culture and practice through their agreements with school districts, Solomon noted. As a health insurer for many school employees, Kaiser Permanente interacts with human resource departments and has a close relationship with union representation. Kaiser Permanente labor management staff works with school employee union representatives to help unions recognize that school and employee wellness is "union business."

As they evaluate Kaiser Permanente's healthy eating and active living interventions, evaluators at the University of California's Nutrition Policy Institute are also helping to refine them.

Resilience in School Environments

The Kaiser Permanente team's experience with the Healthy Schools Program elevated its awareness of influences on learning outcomes that go beyond healthy eating and active living. Childhood adversity can lead to chronic disease and limited life opportunities if it is not addressed, and Kaiser Permanente saw that teachers, administrators, and other school staff had deep concerns about the behavioral health, trauma, and disruptive behavior of their students. These educators were hungry for opportunities to boost social and emotional wellness, improve school climate, and create a positive learning environment for students, teachers, and staff.

"Schools are necessary places to address adversity, toxic stress, and trauma," said Solomon. "If we don't do that, we won't be able to create a positive learning environment and won't be able to prevent chronic disease moving forward."

The Kaiser Permanente team began to focus on supports for students (such as social and emotional learning curricula, positive behavioral skills, and positive discipline). But that wasn't enough—teachers and staff were being left behind. Many felt unprepared to address the trauma their students were experiencing and felt highly stressed themselves as a result. In a baseline survey, 80 percent of school staff said they were affected by traumatic stress and worn out by it.

This tracks with broader national trends; teachers vie with nurses for having the highest stress rate of any occupational group. Some 46 percent of U.S. teachers report daily stress, perhaps helping to explain why as many as half of all teachers leave the profession within their first five years.[28] Alarming on their own terms, those realities result in lost opportunities for them to fully support children. The resilience literature, said Solomon, shows that, while it is not always possible to prevent a child from experiencing adversity, its toxicity can be mitigated by the presence of a trusted adult. "Teachers are in a great position to be that trusted adult, if they're prepared," he said.

Kaiser Permanente launched its Resilience in School Environments (RISE) initiative in 2017 to focus on school staff. [29] Located in 20 schools in four regions, Kaiser Permanente plans to grow its reach to 200 schools by the end of 2019 and 25,000 schools within the next four years through a combination of on-site and virtual interventions.

RISE builds on learnings and evidence from key partner organizations doing leading work in the field: Collaborative Learning for Educational Achievement and Resilience (CLEAR) from Washington State University,[30] and Healthy Environments and Response to Trauma in Schools (HEARTS) from the University of California San Francisco,[31] RISE is designed to build resilience through professional development and by advocating for policy, systems, and environmental changes, with a strong focus on staff wellness. Kaiser Permanente worked with the Los Angeles Education Partnership (LAEP)[32] in the initial 20 schools and is now working with the Alliance for a Healthier Generation as its national scaling partner.

Kaiser Permanente staff is working with these organizations to develop and test a professional development program that incorporates scientific findings about the impact of ACEs and toxic stress on the brains of young children. The intervention trains teachers in classroom management while emphasizing the value of self-care and collective care. (The concept is: "Put on your own oxygen mask before your child's.") Accordingly, the entry point and focus of RISE is on staff/teacher wellness and on supporting school staff to buffer children against trauma and toxic stress.

Our teachers and staff are in this maelstrom and we owe it to them to figure out how to support them to support their students. —Loel Solomon

This effort focuses on policy, practice, and systems change at both the district and school levels. One goal is to build an interdisciplinary team of school leaders who "are prepared to take this resilience work and move it forward," said Solomon. As in the Together for Healthy and Successful Schools initiative, this team may include the school secretary or lunch assistant who has meaningful contact with students and can support their social and emotional wellness.

Among the changes that schools are testing: providing a calm space where teachers can de-stress or take a de-escalating break from conflict situations, creating a buddy system in which a fellow teacher or administrator can take over a classroom during an especially tense period, and offering bereavement leave to teachers after a student is shot. Another piece of the program is ensuring that referrals are in place for children who need a behavioral health specialist or more intensive mental health care.

Evaluating and Scaling RISE

Evaluators from the National Center for School Mental Health at the University of Maryland hope to identify the combination of RISE interventions that drive sought-after outcomes: improving school climate and relationships for staff and students, increasing student attendance and staff retention, and fostering wellness and resilience for staff and students.

Once they do, "We're going to be in scaling mode," said Solomon. The aim will then be to train many other schools in the interventions that work. While the 200 RISE schools will receive intensive resources, Kaiser Permanente is also developing ways to assist the other 14,000-plus schools in its regions. These supports will include workshops, online resources, and professional development around ACEs, trauma, and responding to adversity in a trauma-informed, resilient manner. Kaiser Permanente is also exploring how machine learning and digitally delivered content to build awareness and resilience skills can support this initiative. In time, Kaiser Permanente will explore ways to tie HEAL and RISE efforts together under the Thriving Schools umbrella in order to build synergies between the two efforts and promote student, teacher, and staff health and well-being.

A Final Word

Fostering the connection between education and health is a goal for schools and communities that has the potential to yield positive life outcomes for young people. Yet many schools operate in areas scarred by poverty, violence, poor health, and other difficult circumstances. The children they serve may come to school burdened by stressful experiences at home and in their communities that undermine their development, learning, and health. Although the school has the potential to be a safe haven to help mitigate the toxic stress these experiences generate and prepare children for the future, such schools are themselves hampered by lack of resources and heavy demands from all sides.

This chapter offers models that recognize the whole child and the comprehensive set of supports needed for educational and healthy development—models that also support the health of the teachers and staff who care for children and draw in a wide circle of family and community partners. Although schools and school districts, along with their collaborators, may adapt the models in varying ways, high-need, under-resourced schools and districts will be especially challenged to do so. Yet a comprehensive and holistic approach to educating the whole child is a foundation for success that can benefit all children and youth but most especially—and most necessarily—those young people whose needs are greatest.

5

Employers as Shapers of Health

Roy Ahn, ScD, MPH, Vice President, Public Health, NORC, University of Chicago

Captain Kimberly Elenberg, DNP, MS, Director of Operation Live Well, Office of Personnel Risk & Resiliency, Department of Defense

Ron Z. Goetzel, PhD, Vice President, Consulting and Applied Research, IBM® Watson Health™; Senior Scientist, Director of the Institute for Health and Productivity Studies, Johns Hopkins Bloomberg School of Public Health

Joan C. Williams, JD, Distinguished Professor of Law, Director, Center for WorkLife Law, University of California Hastings College of the Law

Nearly 156 million people age 16 or older were employed in the United States in 2018. More than 128 million worked 35 hours or more per week, and about 27 million worked part-time.[1] Work can offer them income, meaning, friendship, and a sense of community, but it also can generate stress, uncertainty, and feelings of powerlessness. With their significant influence over the lives of their workforce, employers have the authority to make choices that either promote or inhibit a Culture of Health within their organizations. They also may play important roles in building a Culture of Health in the communities in which they are located and where their employees live.

Through its Pioneer Portfolio,[2] its Research on Work, Organization, and Well-Being initiative,[3] and other investments, the Robert Wood Johnson Foundation (RWJF) is committed to promoting understanding of how work can contribute to well-being and equity, and to helping employers apply those insights at their worksites and in their communities. The need is underscored by a 2016 poll commissioned by RWJF in which a significant portion of working adults reported that their current job had an impact on their health.[4] Almost half of those surveyed rated their workplace only fair or poor in its efforts to reduce stress. Most said they go to work when they are sick, and nearly two-thirds said they often or sometimes work overtime or on weekends.

Culture of Health in Practice, Alonzo L. Plough. Oxford University Press (2020) © Robert Wood Johnson Foundation
DOI: 10.1093/oso/9780190071400.001.0001

"Work is a powerful determinant of health," asserted a November 2018 RWJF blog post.[5] Although the future of work is hard to predict, prepare for, or accommodate, many types of employers are taking action to promote health among their employees and within their communities. This chapter examines approaches taken by three of them—Fortune 500 corporations, a large retail chain, and the military.

Roy Ahn explores what Fortune 500 companies tell us, via their public corporate social responsibility reports (also called sustainability reports), about their programs and policies that potentially affect health. Ron Z. Goetzel looks at how efforts by Fortune 500 companies to promote a Culture of Health affect their employees, communities, and their performance in the stock market.

Joan C. Williams analyzes the frontline operations of a large retail apparel chain and illustrates what happens when a company introduces stability and employee control into the work schedules of low-wage sales associates.

Kimberly Elenberg describes the steps a large federal employer, the military, has taken to promote well-being among service members, their families, and the communities in which they live.

Fortune 500 Companies and a Culture of Health

Fortune 500 companies employed 17.5 percent of the U.S. workforce in 2017, according to *Fortune* magazine. These companies generate $12.8 trillion in annual revenue, representing fully two-thirds of the nation's gross domestic product (GDP).[6]

> *Because of their sheer size, the policies and practices of Fortune 500 companies have the potential to affect the health of a broad range of stakeholders. —Roy Ahn*

The recognition that the workplace can make a significant contribution to a Culture of Health, and that corporate health policies have to do more than provide health insurance coverage or offer on-site health or fitness facilities, has drawn the attention of researchers and policymakers in recent years. For their part, many businesses are acting on the knowledge that promoting a healthier workforce can reduce their health care costs, increase productivity, and help them attract skilled workers in an increasingly tight labor market.

By the 1990s and into the 2000s, some companies had realized that "a culture encouraging people to 'do more, work more' doesn't align with people's personal ambitions and their personal needs," said Ron Z. Goetzel, PhD, senior scientist at Johns Hopkins University and vice president at IBM Watson Health.

Corporate Transparency in Reporting
Health-Promoting Activities

Roy Ahn's interest in corporate transparency dates back to his 2005 doctoral dissertation. There, he considered how corporate social performance—defined in the literature as the social responsibility principles, social responsiveness processes, and policies, programs, and observable outcomes that guide the firm's societal relationships[7]—could be used to assess its financial performance and the public health impact of its activities.

"We in public health thought it was prudent that the CDC did not accept money from tobacco companies, for example," Ahn recalls. "But I struggled with how to compare a tobacco company with an insurance company or a company that makes asbestos, when it comes to public impact."

After four years spent analyzing corporate documents, Ahn concluded in his dissertation that most companies did not report about measures that mattered for health. "I figured that a lot of people would care about this," he said. "I was totally wrong." Absent broad interest in his findings, Ahn set the research aside and went on to pursue a career in global maternal health.

Scandals and crises in the early 2000s drew more public attention to corporate transparency, prompting greater interest in public reporting. After the Enron Corporation declared bankruptcy in 2001, for example, more aggressive regulations for reporting on governance were put in place.

Fast-forward to RWJF's launch of its vision for a Culture of Health. Learning of RWJF's commitment and believing that a Culture of Health requires the involvement of large corporations, Ahn retrieved his dissertation and returned to his earlier interests. In his current research, he is looking at which health, well-being, and equity measures are being reported by corporations in their public-facing documents, and which are not.[8]

Ahn's goal is to generate suggestions for greater transparency and identify opportunities to improve reporting. "Part of what I am trying to do is to get people within companies to realize that their health imprint on society doesn't need to be siloed, that there are things that they do and business practices they adopt that affect health in a really profound way." The challenge, he added, is that "many of them don't realize that yet."

Measuring What Corporations Report

Ahn documented the extent of corporate transparency across many types of actions or policies that companies might adopt to promote corporate, employee, and community health. Some, such as health benefits for workers and their families, flexible work policies, leave policies, natural resource use, and product quality, are self-evidently associated with health. Others, such as responsible marketing practices, pricing, financial performance, hiring and promotion, putting women and people of color in leadership positions, and supplier diversity can have health impacts that are less immediately obvious.

A compelling feature of Ahn's study design is the clarity and simplicity of the scoring system, which allows company executives and others to quickly see where they stand on transparency. A score of "0" indicates that an action or policy is not mentioned; a "1" indicates that it is. Supplementary information adds details and nuance about policies that are mentioned.

Ahn selected a random sample of 200 U.S. companies from the 2017 Fortune 500 list. The corporations included in the sample had an average of 62,659 employees. Top industries represented were energy, financials, technology, health care, and transportation.

Findings Point to a Mixed Record

Key findings are based on analyses conducted by Ahn on all 200 companies.

- **Companies frequently reported on their community actions and philanthropic activities, as well as on some of their internal health policies. For example**:
  - More than 98 percent reported on their community philanthropy, such as charitable donations.
  - More than 96 percent reported their natural resource use.
  - About 93 percent reported on their working conditions.
  - At least 80 percent reported on hiring and promotion and product quality.
- **Companies less frequently reported on family-related policies and on some employee- and consumer-related policies. For example**:
  - About 12 percent reported on their downsizing or layoff policies.
  - Just under 20 percent reported on suppliers' social performance.
  - About 22 percent disclosed potential health effects of their products in their marketing material.
  - Less than 40 percent reported on policies related to family medical leave and other forms of leave, dependent care, and pay for low-wage workers.

Some corporations offered examples of strong practices in reporting. For example, JetBlue included detailed information about accidents and safety management; American Express provided extensive information about family medical leave and dependent care policies; and Salesforce.org included detailed information about employee volunteerism.

Opportunities for Public Health Impact

Ahn's study examines only the quality of a company's reporting, not whether the reported policies were actually implemented at the worksite. Nonetheless, his findings suggest opportunities for corporations and the public health sector to work closely together to improve reporting and ultimately address important measures of health and social determinants of health.

One such avenue might be community philanthropy, a centerpiece of corporate reports. "Companies want to talk about how they help society," said Ahn. But the activities they broadcast are not necessarily those with the biggest impact. A company might "spend two pages talking about a $100,000 donation to a local charity," which is likely to be inconsequential in bringing about significant community change, he argues. By contrast, "If an employer like Walmart raises pay for its lowest wage workers by $1 per hour, that change affects millions of people in the United States."

Likewise, Ahn is not convinced that focusing on one or two specific policies should be the priority for corporations. "Ultimately, we need to look at a company's holistic footprint on their stakeholders' health by looking at all of their business practices." Findings from a study published in *JAMA* in April 2019 may lend some support to that perspective. The randomized trial found that employees at worksites with a wellness program were more likely to exercise and manage their weight, but were no more likely to have better clinical indicators of health (e.g., cholesterol levels, blood pressure), health care spending, or employment outcomes.[9] More research is warranted to better understand how workplace wellness policies affect a range of health outcomes and costs. Fuller reporting on all measures is important to understanding these and other factors important to advancing a Culture of Health, Ahn said.

Issues to Watch: Use of Social Media, Employer Role in Climate Change, Workplace Diversity

In a follow-up study funded by RWJF, Ahn is examining how corporations use social media to talk about their health policies.[10] "What you don't get from the static corporate sustainability reports is how people online are reacting to proclamations made by companies," he said. "We are going to see what corporations think is important to tweet about and how much of that is health related."

Ahn identifies two corporate policies that are especially likely to garner attention. First is climate change. Companies already report on their greenhouse gas emissions and carbon offsets, but Ahn suggested that public health and corporate leaders can do much more together to tackle this front-burner issue. (The power of knowledge in helping health systems to act against climate change, and the policies they are implementing to take those actions, are explored in Chapter 10, "The Green Health Care Revolution.")

> *The public health community has to figure out what role they want companies to play in addressing climate change. —Roy Ahn*

The second issue ripe for attention is workplace diversity. Heightened interest in equal pay and equal representation at the executive and board levels is likely to put pressure on companies to be more transparent in these areas.

Do Corporate Investments in Well-Being Pay Off?

Ron Z. Goetzel, PhD, is highly engaged in the worlds of both research and practice. At Johns Hopkins University, he brings academic thinking into business decisions and health and management issues into academia. At IBM' Watson Health™, he develops innovations to help businesses, government agencies, and health care providers optimize their performance by applying data to decision-making.

In opening his presentation at the *Sharing Knowledge* conference, Goetzel noted that publicly held companies whose employees identify them as good places to work, and those with strong track records of employee health programs, perform well in the stock market. For example, the stocks of companies receiving the C. Everett Koop National Health Award (given to companies that demonstrate results both in terms of health impact and economic impact) increased by 325 percent from 2001 to 2014, compared with the market average increase of 105 percent in that period.[11]

Correlation is not causation, however, cautions Goetzel, and many gaps in understanding remain. "It may be that successful companies can afford to attract and retain healthier employees, and then offer gifted workers superior benefits, higher pay, and more amenities," he said.

Based on his experience, Goetzel believes that it will take more than good internal health policies for employers to create a Culture of Health that extends beyond their own walls. It will also require them to become more deeply engaged in the communities in which they are located and where their employees live. Intuition suggests that synergies exist between a company's internal health programs and its programs and activities in communities, but evidence to support that intuition has been lacking. There is insufficient knowledge as well about the extent to which companies that offer in-house programs are those that invest in their communities.

Goetzel sought to narrow both of those gaps.

Measuring Internal and External Health-Building Activities

Most companies agree that workplace health promotion is a good idea, but they are not sure. That's because often they haven't done a good job measuring the programs or the programs are not robust enough to achieve expected outcomes. —Ron Z. Goetzel

Through a partnership between the Johns Hopkins Institute for Health and Productivity Studies and IBM Watson Health, and with support from RWJF, Goetzel's study aimed to determine whether businesses that invest more in employee and community health outperform businesses that invest less.[12]

Goetzel recruited 32 Fortune 500 employers, representing more than 905,000 employees, to find out. Employers came from the retail, manufacturing, health care, education, information, finance, and energy sectors. The measures used were trends in the health risk profiles of employees, medical expenditures, and corporate stock price.

He collected and analyzed four types of data:

- **Employer surveys of internal Culture of Health policies.** To measure what he called an internal Culture of Health, Goetzel looked at worker-focused corporate efforts, such as in-house wellness programs, healthy food offerings, tobacco policies, adequate health insurance coverage, health screenings, flexible work arrangements, senior leadership support, and other indicators.

    A 29-item structured survey was extracted from the Centers for Disease Control and Prevention (CDC) Worksite Health ScoreCard, a tool to help employers assess whether they use evidence-based practices to promote health at their worksites. All 32 employers completed the survey for practices in place in 2013 and again in 2015.

    Survey questions explored the allocation of resources for employee health promotion programs and policies, environmental support for healthy lifestyles, and benefits such as health assessments, in-house exercise facilities, and employee assistance programs.

- **Employer surveys of external Culture of Health policies.** Turning to policies focused on communities where corporations have offices, Goetzel developed measures that he considered indicative of an external Culture of Health. These include charitable donations, meaningful involvement on local boards or coalitions, providing employees with time to volunteer in the community, and marketing support for community health education initiatives.

    Because no evidence-based tool existed to assess contributions to an external Culture of Health, the researchers created one with input from survey and subject matter experts. The 39-item survey covered topics such as resources for community activities, support for employee volunteerism, donations of goods and services, leadership on community boards or coalitions, and involvement in civic issues, such as transportation policy. Twenty-five of the 32 employers completed this survey, also for 2013 and 2015.

- **Employee health risk surveys matched against records of their health expenditures.** Employees of 21 companies reported on nine potentially modifiable health risks (e.g., blood pressure, cholesterol, nutrition, and stress) for 2013 and again for 2015. Health risk and expenditure data came from the IBM MarketScan® Research Databases.
- **Company performance on the S&P 500 index, matched against the overall index.** Researchers collected these data from the 17 publicly traded companies participating in the study, measuring stock performance from January 2013 to August 2017. All 17 companies had completed the internal Culture of Health survey and 14 had completed the external Culture of Health survey.

Driving Down Employee Health Risks, Health Care Utilization, and Cost

- **Employees of companies whose internal Culture of Health scores improved between the two surveys had lower health risks and incurred lower health care costs.**
  - Employees who were high risk in 2013 saw significant risk reduction in 2015 for four of the nine risks: body mass index (BMI), blood pressure, nutrition, and tobacco use.
  - For three of the nine risk factors—nutrition, depression, and alcohol use—employees who were not at risk in 2013 were at even lower risk for the same factor in 2015.
  - Both at-risk and not-at-risk employees reported increased risk for stress in 2015.
  - At-risk and not-at-risk employees filled fewer drug prescriptions over the two years and the growth in their health care expenditures slowed, but not significantly.
- **Health risks and health care costs were reduced, but to a limited degree, for employees of companies whose external Culture of Health scores improved.**
  - For three of the nine risk factors—cholesterol, glucose levels, and tobacco use—employees at risk in 2013 were less likely to be at risk in 2015. However, they were again at greater risk for stress.
  - Employees who did not face the risks associated with BMI and stress in 2013 were less likely to be at risk for those factors in 2015. However,

employees who did not face risks associated with depression and stress, respectively, were at greater risk for these factors in 2015.
- There was a significant reduction in hospital admission and emergency department visits, but expenditures slowed only minimally over two years.

Associations With Stock Performance

- **Employers with improved internal Culture of Health scores outperformed the S&P 500 index, while those with lower scores underperformed the index.**
  - The nine companies with improved internal Culture of Health scores during the study period saw a 115 percent increase in their stock prices from 2013 to 2017. The S&P 500 index grew by 69 percent during that time.
  - The eight companies whose scores did not improve realized a stock price increase of only 43 percent in those years.
- **Surprisingly, employers with improved external Culture of Health scores underperformed the S&P 500 index, while those with lower scores outperformed the index.**
  - The seven companies with improved external Culture of Health scores saw only a 44 percent growth in stock performance, compared with 69 percent growth of the index.
  - The seven companies whose scores did not improve achieved an 89 percent increase in stock performance.

Details of the study methods and findings appear in the *Journal of Occupational and Environmental Medicine*[13,14] and the *American Journal of Health Promotion.*[15]

Next Steps

There are 150 million Americans who go to work every day, and their employers can play a major role in improving the lives of those workers. —
Ron Z. Goetzel

Investing in employee health at the worksite has a measurable payoff, concluded Goetzel. Higher scores on internal Culture of Health policies yielded results that matter to large employers, including better employee health and robust stock performance. Tools exist to guide companies in taking actions to promote a Culture of Health for their employees, and if employers are committed to doing so, this strategy is ripe for expansion.

Corporate investments in building an external Culture of Health, however, are inadequately studied or understood and should be a priority area for researchers, corporate leaders, and public health professionals, urged Goetzel. "Most employers don't know what an external Culture of Health looks like. They don't know how to create it, how to measure it, or what its effect might be."

Perhaps, he suggested, benefits from investments in internal health show up more quickly. Factors such as poverty rates or access to health care might have a stronger influence on community health, but interventions to address them are hard to implement and scale in the short term. That could be especially true if the "dose" of a community investment is diluted because the company invests across a wide territory.

A first step in better understanding corporate investments to promote an external Culture of Health might be refining a survey instrument comparable to the well-established CDC Worksite Health ScoreCard, Goetzel suggested. There is no equivalent tool to measure external Culture of Health policies, and although Goetzel's team undertook a rigorous process to create one, their tool is new and relatively untested.

A second step could be to look more closely at the organizational units within a company responsible for promoting health and well-being. Goetzel found little correlation in scores on internal and external investments, possibly because internal health policies tend to fall under the purview of human resources departments, while external policies likely fall within community relations or external affairs. "Internal and external initiatives to promote a Culture of Health are not coordinated and are often performed by different company divisions with separate goals and outcomes of interest," he observed.

What Does It Really Mean for Corporations to Promote Health?

Noting the complementary nature of their studies, Goetzel and Ahn engaged in a vigorous conversation with each other and with attendees at the *Sharing Knowledge* breakout session. Questions about the tension between a company's products or services and its employment policies dominated much of the discussion.

Might a company that sells products that some people find objectionable nonetheless offer progressive hiring, promotion, benefit, leave, and wellness policies to its employees? How should public health professionals weigh this tension? How should investors consider it? Should there be public health standards about acceptable corporate behavior in this area, or are these personal decisions best made by individuals?

When the nature of a company's products first began to draw public attention, the focus was primarily through an investment lens. "It used to be that mutual funds—socially minded mutual funds—would rate companies as being good or bad based on a few metrics—military arms, pornography, tobacco, or alcohol," Ahn explained. Those ratings would then be used to screen certain companies out of their portfolios.

But the issues involved are often more nuanced and complex, commented several audience members. One offered the example of a bank that releases employees to volunteer in their communities and offers good internal wellness programs but has a poor track record of lending in communities of color. It was unclear whether that would show up in corporate reports or on measures used by socially concerned funds.

"Bad" and "good" products and services fall along a spectrum, Goetzel acknowledged. "Companies that produce tobacco or firearms may be easily identifiable as producing 'bad' public health outcomes when handled irresponsibly," he said. Other companies, such as pharmaceuticals, produce products that provide social benefit, but some may be priced out of reach. "This is a complex area that requires ethicists as well as public policy experts to weigh in."

Ahn believes that "if you focus on how companies make their money—their policies and priorities—rather than how they give it away—their charitable donations and community activities—you will have a more sensitive barometer of impact." He also suggested taking a community-wide perspective on a company's involvement in health. RWJF's *County Health Rankings & Roadmaps*, for example, offers important data and insights on how some communities, including the corporations that operate within them, take steps to promote an external Culture of Health and reduce health disparities.

Ahn suggests developing a public health scorecard to identify corporate policies that promote well-being. Available to the public, it would allow individuals to weigh their concerns about what a company sells against what it offers its employees and communities as they consider their consumer purchases and investment decisions. "One angle is to put the data out there and let people decide for themselves, based on what they believe is important," he said.

> *If you believe that paying a living wage is very important, for example, you might weigh that more heavily than other factors, such as the products a company makes or other employment practices. —Roy Ahn*

Responding to a question about tracking employer policies toward low- and moderate-income workers, Ahn noted that scorecards and transparency also allow within-industry comparisons. "If you can get one company within an industry to move on something, the others naturally have to follow. I see that as a practical benefit of a scorecard."

Returning to an earlier comment by Goetzel, another lively discussion centered on the dose of a corporate investment. Companies with a presence in scores or hundreds of communities may make a substantial overall commitment, but that commitment might touch so many places that it has little effect on any one of them. As a result, companies might not realize the results they had hoped for and could become discouraged from further giving. More research and fine-tuning could shed light on how dose influences the value of an investment.

A final discussion centered on what happens when corporations that invest in wellness programs to reduce stress or build resiliency among employees also have a corporate culture that undermines those very programs. Cultures characterized by inflexible work schedules, expectations that employees will work long hours, or poor management practices undermine internal wellness programs, argued one audience member. Wellness programs and employment policies may conflict, agreed Goetzel, again noting that they tend to fall under the purview of different and possibly uncoordinated departments.

Ahn hopes for a data center that collects publicly reported corporate data on social determinants of health. It would be "a big place," he said, "where public health researchers could analyze the data, where management researchers could analyze the data, and where companies . . . could have all of the social and environmental data in one place as well, to streamline their reporting functions."

Stable Scheduling, Worker Productivity, and Retail Sales

Narrowing to a single sector of the American economy, Joan C. Williams, JD, director of the Center for WorkLife Law at the University of California Hastings College of the Law, examined the issue of stable scheduling in the retail industry.

Brick-and-mortar retail stores remain an important part of American life, despite the growth of internet commerce. They employ nearly 16 million people—more than 10 percent of the nation's workforce—and include companies as large as Walmart and as small as a local hardware store.[16]

Although retail stores struggle to compete with internet sales in their prices and range of offerings, their competitive edge comes from delivering a high-quality shopping experience in which customers leave the store with a product they feel is right for them, Williams said. Retaining this edge requires the presence of well-trained, engaged sales associates who know the inventory, can locate products, are current on promotions and specials, and have time to keep shelves stocked and stores tidy.

Much is expected of these workers, but little is offered to support them in return. Median annual earnings for full-time retail workers were $31,980, according to a 2017 report from the Bureau of Labor Statistics,[17] but a survey of retail workers found that 47 percent of them work only part-time and earn considerably less.[18] A study of younger retail worker schedules found that 87 percent reported schedule fluctuations that affected, on average, 48 percent of their weekly hours; 50 percent reported receiving their schedules with notice of a week or less; and 44 percent said their employer alone determined the timing of their work.[19]

Not surprisingly, sales associates working in these situations report that it is difficult to secure child care, participate in school and community activities, or take on second jobs to help make ends meet. Numerous studies have documented the negative effects of volatile schedules on the well-being of workers, while other research confirms that employees' well-being improves when they are able to plan and predict their work hours. Yet the problem persists, and stable schedules remain the exception among retail sales associates.

Williams introduced her study by pointing to problems inherent in applying the "just in time, or lean, scheduling" model to retail stores. Lean scheduling, designed to minimize business expenses by keeping labor and inventory costs as low as possible, she noted, has yielded efficiencies in manufacturing but is a flawed model when applied to a sector that relies heavily on people.

Retail scheduling this way has been rationalized as a means of accommodating changes in customer traffic due to poor weather forecasts, in-store promotions, or other fluid factors, or to meet aggressive end-of-month revenue targets. But the hidden costs have been well documented—messy stores, no one available to help customers, long checkout lines, high turnover, and low employee engagement. Yet these are rarely factored into scheduling algorithms.

A "myopic mindset" causes retailers to spend billions of dollars on advertisements to drive customers into stores, and yet embrace labor practices that undermine the stores' ability to turn that traffic into sales. — Joan C. Williams

The Stable Scheduling Study

With support from RWJF's *Evidence for Action* signature research program and other funders, Williams set out to learn whether schedules of retail sales associates could be made more stable without hurting store revenues, and the Stable Scheduling Study got under way.[20] "We wanted to change an ecosystem in which many practices intersect to undermine stability," she said.

Officials at Gap Inc., a global retailer with six chains of clothing stores and 135,000 employees, agreed to participate as partners. The study was "the first randomized controlled trial of a multi-component intervention designed to shift schedules in hourly retail jobs toward greater stability," Williams noted.

Listening to Workers

Prior research by Williams's colleague and co-principal investigator Susan J. Lambert, PhD, associate professor at the University of Chicago School of Social Service Administration, identified four priority areas for improvement: more *consistency* in shift starting and ending times, more *predictability* that hours worked aligned with scheduled hours, increased *worker input and control* of their schedules, and modest improvements in the *adequacy* of hours scheduled.

The study team, which also included co–principal investigator Saravanan Kesavan, DBA, TOM, associate professor and Sarah Graham Kenan Scholar at the University of North Carolina, began by listening to store managers and sales associates talk about the scheduling changes they most wanted. Three San Francisco Bay Area Gap stores pilot-tested seven specific changes from March through October 2015. By the end of the pilot, Gap management was convinced of the value of two of them, which they then introduced nationwide: a policy requiring that schedules be published two weeks in advance, and a prohibition against canceling schedules with as little as two hours' notice before a shift began.

Gap retail outlets in the Bay Area and in Chicago participated in the full study from November 2015 through August 2016: 19 stores were randomly selected as treatment sites and nine served as controls. The treatment stores were urged, but not required—what Williams calls "a randomized encouragement design"—to implement the remaining five changes suggested by store staff:

- **Stable shift structure:** Standardizing storewide shift start and end times (consistency)
- **Core scheduling:** Assigning associates the same days and hours of work from week to week (predictability)
- **Technology-enabled shift swapping:** A mobile app allowing managers to post additional shifts and workers to swap shifts among themselves (worker input and control)
- **Part-time plus:** Giving core sales associates a guarantee of 20 or more hours of work each week (adequacy)
- **Targeted additional staff:** Adding staffing allocations for certain times of the week at no cost to the store budget (adequacy)

Quantitative data came from personnel records, time clock records, shift schedules posted by managers, detailed sales figures, records of store traffic, and records of all shifts posted and picked up on the mobile app.

Qualitative data included manager surveys; pre- and post-intervention surveys of employees about their health, well-being, and commitment to the store; manager interviews; and focus groups with sales associates.

Stable Scheduling Makes a Difference

> *We found that shifting to more schedule stability isn't good only for sales associates—it is good for business, too. —Joan C. Williams*

- **Modest but significant improvements were seen in consistency, predictability, and worker input and control.** Adequacy of work hours did not increase significantly.
  - **Consistency:** The odds of an associate working the same day of the week were 25 percent in treatment stores but only 20 percent in control stores. Improvements in consistency also increased on-time arrivals of associates. "Knowing that their shift is going to be the same week to week, they know what time to leave, what buses to take," reported one store manager.
  - **Predictability:** Associates in treatment stores were better able to predict their work hours—71 percent said they could easily anticipate how many hours they would work, compared with 63 percent of associates in control stores. Associates with predictable schedules delivered better customer service, according to their managers. A sales associate on a core schedule "is here so often she knows where the product is, and she's able to tell you if we have something or don't," commented one manager.
  - **Worker input and control:** Most associates (62%) posted or picked up a shift using the app, including 70 percent of associates under age 21 and 46 percent of associates over age 50.
  - **Adequacy:** Adequacy of work hours did not increase for the average associate, but it did for "part-time plus" associates. Those associates worked 26 hours per week, compared with 21 hours per week before they were given the scheduling guarantee. These associates were also more likely to be older and have more seniority than other associates.
- **Modest improvements in shift stability delivered notable improvements in business outcomes in participating stores without drawing traffic away from other Gap stores in the area.** Williams attributed improvements to "higher conversion rates," meaning a higher proportion of visitors purchased goods, and improved "basket values," meaning more purchases per customer.

- Median sales in treatment stores increased by 7 percent during the nine-month study period, in an industry that aims for increases of just 1 percent to 2 percent annually. Productivity increased 5 percent, translating to $6.20 of new revenue per hour of labor.
- Treatment stores earned an average of $4,363 per week more than control stores, yielding an estimated $2.9 million in increased revenues for Gap during the study period.
- **Much of the instability came from corporate headquarters policies rather than from changes in store traffic**.
  - Only 30 percent of schedule fluctuation could be attributed to changes in anticipated customer traffic resulting from weather, store promotions, and other local conditions.
  - Much of the remaining 70 percent of fluctuation likely came from headquarters-generated actions, according to store managers. They noted last-minute changes in shipment dates or number of product units, last-minute changes in promotions, and visits to stores by corporate executives as primary sources of instability.

Study findings were reported in popular and professional media, including the *New York Times*,[21] *Harvard Business Review*,[22, 23] and *Slate*.[24] The final report appears on the Center for WorkLife Law website.[25]

Although not a direct outcome of the study, Walmart subsequently adopted two of the study's interventions: core scheduling and tech-enabled shift swapping. "There are a lot of people affected by this change, and it is also a kind of seal of approval for the findings," Williams said.

Improvements in Sales Don't Necessarily Drive Change

Williams underscored the remarkable nature of a relatively easy strategy to increase retail sales in the range of 7 percent at a time when it has been hard for the industry to raise revenues. "The importance of that finding cannot be overestimated," she emphasized.

But just because the business case for stable scheduling is well established, that "is not where the action is," she warned. Achieving shift stability requires changes in management practice so that headquarters staff from human resources, finance, information technology, field operations, and other departments work in collaboration with store managers to address the multiple causes of instability.

What is holding organizations back now, according to Williams, is the change management challenge. "Effecting a change to more stable scheduling is a complex process that requires leadership from the top and the involvement of many different people in the organization, all of them using systems designed to pro-duce instability, not stability," she said. "That is a totally different topic than producing evidence that there are business benefits to be had."

Lessons for Researchers

The stable scheduling study benefited from the support of a Gap executive who had access to a budget and to store managers, and the authority to make decisions. Williams also noted the essential role of front-line managers "who can tell you what is actually going to work and what will not work in a brutally honest fashion."

The other key to success is to insist that the company appoint an internal project manager charged with interacting with the study team and getting them what they need. Then, she noted, "You fly under the radar screen, so you don't have to go back and get authority all over again when personnel changes at the company."

> *What three professors and a score of graduate students found is what every store manager already knew. You don't know their business as well as they do, so listen to them.* —Joan C. Williams

Fostering Health and Well-Being in the Military

The Department of Defense (DoD), and indeed the country, need a fit, healthy, and ready armed services force. Captain Kimberly Elenberg, DNP, MS, is working hard to make that happen. With 24 years as an active-duty officer, her passion for building a Culture of Health within the DoD is fueled by her belief that all young people should be healthy enough to choose to enlist. When med-ical and social determinants of health preclude those choices, they eliminate a source of employment that would otherwise offer people training, benefits, and career opportunities.

> *Broadening the pool of recruits is a DoD priority. Efforts that address the social determinants of health not only for service members living on bases, but also for current and future members living in communities, helps build a sustainable force.* —Kimberly Elenberg

The foundational strength of the DoD is its nearly 2.87 million members, in-cluding its 732,079 civilian employees.[26] The Total Force includes nearly

1.3 million people on active duty in the Army, Navy, Air Force, Marine Corps, and Coast Guard, and 1.1 million in the Coast Guard Reserve, the National Guard, and other reserve forces.[27] Reserve Component and National Guard members are generally required to meet military physical and cognitive readiness standards while working civilian jobs in communities.

The DoD is also one of America's largest employers, making military personnel a critical component of the nation's workforce. Service personnel are trained to de-escalate crises, engage in battle and peacekeeping missions around the world, and cope with natural disasters at home. Forces may be called up at a moment's notice and for unspecified periods of time.

Most Americans agree that attending to the well-being of these service members and investing in the development of healthy, capable future recruits should be national priorities. Maintaining a robust and well-supported force that reflects America's diverse population is a shared responsibility of the DoD, other federal and state agencies, and the companies that employ service members and their families in communities across the country. Yet challenges persist in living up to these responsibilities.

In 2017, 71 percent of all Americans ages 17 to 24 would have been ineligible to serve in the military, many of them because of physical health limitations.[28] Survey data from the Centers for Disease Control and Prevention suggest that by 2030, nearly 64 percent of potential recruits may not qualify for service due to their weight.

Military Personnel Face Health Challenges

For many, the ability to serve brings purpose, meaning, and a sense of comradery, but it also can generate stress, uncertainty, and at times, financial strain. About 70 percent of active military personnel live off base, many earning only modest salaries in their communities. Often, it is difficult for a military spouse to find a job that generates a needed second income, given that the family may have to relocate. Reservists who also hold civilian jobs struggle with the same wage and benefit concerns as the rest of the workforce. The combination of all these factors perhaps makes it unsurprising that active service members and their families used $43 million in Supplemental Nutrition Assistance Program (SNAP) and Special Supplemental Nutrition Program for Women, Infants, and Children (WIC) benefits in Fiscal Year (FY) 2015.

Like their civilian peers, service members strive to find healthy ways to balance work and personal activities, but they have the added responsibility of meeting enhanced military readiness requirements. With only limited exceptions, the ability to deploy is a condition of employment in the military. Service personnel who cannot achieve or maintain fitness or body fat standards are at amplified risk for nonbattle injuries: the most common nonbattle causes of hospitalization among service members unable to complete their deployment are mental health conditions and musculoskeletal injuries.

Elenberg believes that a more intentional approach to health maintenance of service members within the military is essential, and she draws an analogy to the system for routine maintenance that is used for ships, tanks, and other equipment. "We can project that a given piece of equipment will require maintenance and need new parts within a given period of time," she said. There is no equivalent system for personnel, she added. "We assess an individual's medical readiness to deploy, but if we can estimate the likelihood that the recruit will complete the deployment and integrate well back into the community, we will help service members succeed and reinforce unit cohesion. We must consider the fact that humans need maintenance too."

If we are really going to change the culture in the DoD, we need to start thinking as much about people and maintaining people as we do about maintaining equipment. —Kimberly Elenberg

Aligning the Military Health Agenda With the Culture of HealthAction Framework

Given its influence over the lives of its workforce, DoD is striving to promote a Culture of Health within the service and to build external partnerships that will shape a Culture of Health in the communities where current and potential service members live. Moving away from a narrow clinical view of illness and injury and toward a holistic view that wellness is based on the integration of mind, body, and spirit, in 2011 the Joint Chiefs of Staff created Total Force Fitness,[29] a strategy to understand, assess, and maintain service members' well-being and to sustain their ability to carry out missions.

Through Total Force Fitness, Elenberg works with teams of leaders from within and outside the services, including academic institutions and nongovernmental organizations. "We must capitalize on our strengths to effectively address challenges that none of us can adequately tackle on our own," she explained.

RWJF proved a natural ally in this effort. Elenberg aligned the DoD Total Force Fitness initiative, which addresses individual "Total Force Domains" of physical, social, behavioral, environmental, medical, dental, and spiritual health,[30] with the broader perspective featured in RWJF's Culture of Health Action Framework. The synergy between the individually focused Total Force Fitness framework and the community and systems-focused Culture of Health Action Framework served as a launchpad for Building Healthy Military Communities.

> *I liked that the Action Framework was action-oriented, and that equity was depicted as part of all the Action Areas. —Kimberly Elenberg*

Building Healthy Military Communities

Despite some differences, the military shares many of the challenges that Goetzel, Ahn, and Williams identify in the private sector. Emergency deployments, for example, create scheduling volatility similar to what Williams describes in retail environments. The DoD has a stake in promoting transparency and an internal and external Culture of Health, just as Ahn and Goetzel report in their studies of Fortune 500 companies. The military also shares the problems of siloed decision-making and inadequate coordination that Goetzel noted.

Elenberg oversees one initiative that aims to address these kinds of challenges. Started in 2016, Building Healthy Military Communities is a multiyear pilot program to examine and address barriers to health and service readiness among military personnel and their families who live off base.[31] Using a tool for aggregating publicly reported health indicators, DoD identified high-risk counties in seven states with large military populations—Florida, Indiana, Maryland, Minnesota, Mississippi, New Mexico, and Oklahoma—for the pilot.

The three-phase initiative is designed to promote a Culture of Health for everyone, whether or not they serve in the military. It involves: (1) a qualitative and quantitative analysis of health, demographic, and other conditions in each pilot site; (2) the development of Building Healthy Military Communities state action plans that align with existing state health and economic improvement plans and priorities aimed at all residents; and (3) evaluations of interventions undertaken under the state action plans. Participants from local, county, and state agencies convene as state teams to design and implement plans in each site. A member of the military serves as the Building Healthy Military Communities state coordinator in each location, bringing an essential military perspective to community partners.

State team advisory groups comprising executive-level government, non-profit, and private officials oversee plan development and implementation and promote connections across sites. They also serve as a link between DoD staff and public health experts at each location. Mental illness, substance misuse, obesity, physical inactivity, access to quality child care, and unemployment are typically shared concerns.

Some Early Observations

Outcome data from Building Healthy Military Communities are not yet available, but Elenberg noted some promising responses. Among issues being addressed is the fact that military families sometimes underutilize state and community resources, frequently because program intake protocols targeted only veterans while overlooking current service members. In at least one pilot site in Oklahoma, social service agency staff began asking applicants about their current as well as prior military service.

Another challenge is that reserve corps members have in recent years been required to participate in more days of drills and trainings, which means more time away from their regular jobs. One company in Minnesota has implemented a pay differential for members who would otherwise have lost wages while attending drills and training.

Still another promising approach is one taken by San Juan College, a two-year community college in New Mexico, which established fast-track programs to provide formal training and the certifications that are required for civilian employment to service members and others. In 2019, the college added interest and aptitude testing, wraparound support services to help students succeed, and training in resume preparation and job interviewing skills.

> Our intended outcome is for other public health professionals to use Building Healthy Military Communities as an exemplar for establishing diverse and effective partnerships to address psychosocial determinants of health. — Kimberly Elenberg

A Final Word

The narratives in this chapter describe various efforts to enhance the contribution that large employers—Fortune 500 companies, retail chains, and the military—can make to a Culture of Health and to promoting health equity. Although they differ in many ways, these stories converge on one important insight: the workplace is a social determinant of health. Importantly, health is not the purview of human resources or any other single entity, but rather is shaped by an ecosystem that involves human resources, finance, legal, operations, and many other departments.

SECTION III

CHALLENGING INEQUITY THROUGH SYSTEMS INNOVATION

To break down barriers to a Culture of Health and achieve true health equity, the nation must confront persistent structural challenges in marginalized communities, which are often communities of color. Fortunately, policymakers, academics, practitioners, and advocates are paying considerable attention to the urban and rural areas still haunted by poverty, violence, and neglect.

People who have historically been excluded from decision-making also are coming to the table as they become empowered to develop solutions that fit their own needs and the needs of their communities. Novel responses are being designed, implemented, and evaluated as the drive for innovation picks up speed. It will take effort, dedication, resources, and time to move forward—and views on how this should happen diverge widely. Progress may be slow, but progress is being made.

Recognizing that the United States has the highest rate of incarceration among all nations in the world, "Disrupting the Cycle of Incarceration" examines the root causes for the trend and its health-damaging consequences. Contributors describe both broad-based solutions and targeted local efforts to break the cycle of incarceration at various points: before arrest, within prison walls, after release, and across genera-tions. Changing the narrative is a feature of many efforts, as activists find new ways to talk about poverty, crime, and prison, and adults with a his-tory of incarceration commit to renewing bonds with their children.

"The Opioid Epidemic: Busting Myths and Sharing Solutions" tackles the unprecedented public health crisis of opioid addiction and deaths by overdose. The chapter's contributors describe the patterns of the epidemic, with a Spotlight on rural addiction; dispel myths; and talk about the evidence for actions that lower rates of addiction and overdose. They also offer glimmers of hope from states that are targeting both the supply of opioids and the demand for them with creative "whole community" approaches, shifting away from the criminal justice system, providing better access to treatment, and crafting innovative reimbursement strategies.

Exchanging rhetoric for factual information, "Achieving Health Equity for Immigrants and Their Children" opens with a data-based portrait of immigrants in America. Nearly 44 million immigrants live in the United States (13.5% of the population),[1] and their health, and that of their children, is directly affected by their legal status and by U.S. policy. Public policy at both the federal and state levels—including Deferred Action for Childhood Arrivals (DACA), changes in "public charge" rules, and eligibility for driver's licenses and prenatal care—are all significant influences on health status and access to care.

Adverse environmental conditions resulting from climate change and human-made disasters are an increasingly serious health threat, especially to disenfranchised, vulnerable, and indigenous populations. "Climate Change, Environmental Stressors, and Resilience" looks at the immediate effects and aftermath of disasters, drawing on examples that include Hurricane Maria in Puerto Rico, Superstorm Sandy in the Brooklyn neighborhood of Sunset Park, and the *Exxon Valdez* oil spill in Alaska. The potential for community resilience is a bright spot among these challenges, especially where a commitment to social justice becomes the foundation for responding to the social and economic shocks associated with environmental catastrophes.

As a major producer of pollution, the health care sector is a significant contributor to climate change. But as "The Green Health Care Revolution" documents, a movement to reduce the industry's carbon footprint has gained momentum. Strategies to reduce many sources of pollution are targeted at multiple corners of the industry: energy consumption, "green bond" financing, operating-room-generated greenhouse gases, hospital waste, and more. Despite formidable challenges, support for greening health care is building.

The final chapter, "Driving Innovation Through Medicaid," highlights the expanding use of Medicaid to address social determinants of health, particularly housing instability and opioid addiction. With one in five Americans participating in Medicaid,[2] the program has the reach and influence to play a key role in promoting health and health equity, especially through research and demonstration waivers that allow states to experiment. The chapter's contributors offer examples of innovative programming and service delivery in three states and spotlight a major insurer's commitment to address the root causes of homelessness among its Medicaid beneficiaries.

The topics explored in these chapters are sometimes viewed as intractable, "wicked" problems that are difficult, if not impossible, to fix. Difficult they are, but resourceful and imaginative individuals and organizations continue to pursue innovative solutions that can help move all in America ever closer to a Culture of Health.

Disrupting the Cycle of Incarceration

Rev. Juard Barnes, Midwest Regional Director, Faith in Action

Devlin Hanson, PhD, Senior Research Associate, Center on Labor, Human Services, and Population, Urban Institute

Jim Parsons, MSc, Vice President and Research Director, Vera Institute of Justice

Harold Pollack, PhD, Helen Ross Professor, School of Social Service Administration, University of Chicago, and Co-Director, University of Chicago Crime Lab

Vance Simms, Founder/Executive Director, Father Matters

Teresa Eckrich Sommer, PhD, Research Associate Professor, Institute for Policy Research, Northwestern University

The United States, with just 4.4 percent of the world's population, has about 22 percent of the world's incarcerated people and the world's highest incarceration rate.[1] Reducing incarceration levels, particularly in communities of color and disadvantage, is a vital building block of a Culture of Health.

How do we prevent people from being incarcerated in the first place? What effect does incarceration have on the health of individuals and communities? How do we ensure that incarcerated people do not return to their communities with more physical, mental, and social health challenges than when they left? How do we help formerly incarcerated individuals find stable housing and employment, renew and strengthen family ties, and establish the supports they need to stay out of prison?

The contributors to this chapter offer some answers to those questions. After an overview by Jim Parsons, they describe four interventions designed to disrupt the incarceration cycle. Parsons looks at efforts by the Vera Institute of Justice to transform conditions of confinement for young adults held in prison, while Teresa Eckrich Sommer assesses "two-generation" approaches that help young children and their parents find surer footing. Devlin Hanson examines

Culture of Health in Practice, Alonzo L. Plough. Oxford University Press (2020) © Robert Wood Johnson Foundation
DOI: 10.1093/oso/9780190071400.001.0001

the role of supportive housing in breaking the homelessness–jail–homelessness cycle, and Harold Pollack reports on a Chicago program that connects police and mental health providers in order to prevent the arrest of low-level drug offenders.

Juard Barnes then talks more broadly about changing the narrative on poverty, crime, and incarceration as he describes a successful campaign to rework plans for a new criminal justice center. Finally, a chapter Spotlight describes Vance Simms and Father Matters, a mentoring program that helps fathers get their lives back on track and develop more satisfying relationships with their children.

A Profile of Mass Incarceration

Some 2.2 million people are incarcerated in federal and state prisons and local jails in the United States, an increase of 500 percent over the last 40 years.[2] (Prisons are designed for long-term sentences; jails hold people pretrial and for short stays, averaging 24 days.) That represents 860 people per 100,000 adults aged 18 and older.[3] Another 840,000 people are on parole (early supervised release from prison), and 3.7 million are on probation (generally a prison sentence alternative).[4]

Although incarceration rates are at their lowest level in two decades, the steady rise from 1980 to 2008 is "unprecedented in U.S. history and internationally," said Jim Parsons of the Vera Institute of Justice. Mass incarceration grew out of laws enacted from the 1970s through the 1990s as part of the so-called war on drugs. Focused particularly on communities of color, these laws mandated longer prison sentences and compulsory incarceration for multiple minor offenses. One in five prisoners now serve time for a drug offense.

Yet after peaking in the early 1990s, violent crime and property crime fell by about half between 1993 and 2017.[5] "This idea that all those people are behind bars because of lots of crime is entirely unfounded," Parsons stressed. Incarceration, not crime, is the issue.

Race Is a Dominant Factor in Incarceration Rates

In 1871, the Supreme Court of Virginia drew a line from slavery to prison when it defined the incarcerated person as "the slave of the state," a characterization that led to horrific practices in the treatment of prisoners, especially black men, that lasted into the 20th century and continues in the racialization of the criminal justice system to this day.[6]

People of color are far more likely to be incarcerated than are whites, with blacks 5.9 times more likely and Hispanics 3.1 times more likely.[7] And in a nation where blacks represent 13 percent of the total population, they constitute 33 percent of the prison and 34 percent of the jail populations. Overall, people from racial and ethnic minority groups represent 60 percent of the incarcerated population, yet represent only 39 percent of the nation's total population.

A national conversation about racism and race and the criminal justice system is really important. —*Jim Parsons*

Incarceration is Concentrated in Disadvantaged Communities— those characterized by poverty, unemployment, family disruption, and racial isolation

In the East Harlem section of New York City, incarceration rates are 302 per 100,000 people; next door, in the more affluent Upper East Side, the rate is 15 per 100,000.[8] And the increased incarceration is not only a result of increased crime. Among communities with similar crime rates, those with high concentrations of disadvantage experienced incarceration rates that were more than three times higher than those with less disadvantage.[9]

Incarceration Is Increasingly Rural

Over half of the prison and jail population in the United States is from small towns and rural areas, with incarceration rates in those areas increasing at a time when metropolitan, urban, and suburban rates have remained flat or decreased.[10] Concentrated poverty, industrial decline, the opioid epidemic, and other factors all contribute to this trend. (The characteristics and challenges of rural communities that result in higher rates of incarceration, as well as opportunities to reverse troubling trends, are explored in greater depth in Chapter 3, "Pathways to Change in Rural America.")

Female Incarceration Rates Are Rising Faster than Male Incarceration Rates

Between 1978 and 2015, the population in women's state prisons grew by 834 percent, more than twice the rate of increase in the male prison population.[11] In 26 states, female incarceration rates exceed those of any other country.[12] Yet criminal justice reform efforts in many states have ignored women's incarceration.

Children of Incarcerated Parents Are at Special Risk

Studies have found paternal incarceration to be clearly harmful to children. Some research directly links maternal incarceration to poor outcomes for children, while other findings suggest these outcomes result from risk factors present prior to a mother's incarceration.[13,14] (See "Spotlight: Fathers Mentoring Fathers" for a look at a program that helps formerly incarcerated fathers pull their lives together and reconnect with their kids.)

Strategies for Change

Addressing mass incarceration in the United States requires a range of approaches and tactics that target multiple levels of the complex criminal justice system. Jim Parsons offered three strategies that a society serious about driving long-term change should consider.

Focus on Multiple Jurisdictional Levels

State prisons house the majority of incarcerated individuals (about 1.3 million), followed by county or city jails (about 741,000).[15] Jails have a particularly significant impact on local communities because people enter jails 10.6 million times each year.[16] Federal prisons, the focus of reform legislation passed by Congress in December 2018, house just 181,000 people.[17]

The systems that move people into prisons and jails also operate at many jurisdictional levels, including courts, which tend to be organized at the state level, and police departments, which are mostly local. "We need to focus on all these levels of jurisdiction if we are going to address the issue of mass incarceration," emphasized Parsons.

Rethink the Front End of the Criminal Justice System

The time may be right for "a fundamental rethinking of how the front end of the justice system operates and how we respond to societal behaviors which are based in lack of resources, poverty, and ill health," said Parsons. Strategies that support this rethinking include:

- Reducing or eliminating cash bail so that people do not spend pretrial time in jail only because they cannot afford to pay cash bail. People going to trial from jail are more likely to be given prison or jail sentences than those people who have spent pretrial time out on bail.[18]

- Implementing programs in which police officers refer people to mental health and social services as alternatives to arrest. Mental health crises, homelessness, and substance use disorders are among the many situations better suited to community-based interventions.
- Addressing the number of people in prison or jail because they failed to comply with conditions of community supervision (probation or parole).

Reduce the Sentences of People Convicted of Violent Crimes

Addressing mass incarceration by focusing only on people who have committed low-level, nonviolent offenses tends to have public appeal, but 55 percent of people in state prisons have been convicted of a violent crime, with associated long sentences.[19] Even if everyone imprisoned for a nonviolent offense were released, the U.S. incarceration rate would still exceed that of most other countries.

Long sentences are often unnecessary for public safety, given that people are much less likely to commit crimes as they age, and long sentences rarely make fiscal sense, given the cost of prison operations. Yet the number of incarcerated individuals 55 years of age or older increased 280 percent between 1999 and 2016,[20] making this demographic one of the main drivers of the prison population size. Moreover, when people who have been incarcerated for a long time are released, they are likely to bring home the problems they experienced in prison and to be poorly prepared to reintegrate into the community.

"We need to think differently about how we deal with violence," Parsons said.

Mass Incarceration and Public Health

Mass incarceration is a population-level driver of health and needs to be considered on the same level as diet, exercise, and smoking. Criminal justice system involvement is of the same order. —Jim Parsons

Health in Prison

People often enter prison or jail in poor health, which tends to worsen while they are there. Incarcerated people have substantially higher rates of substance use disorders, AIDS, hepatitis C, HIV, and tuberculosis than the general population. Rates of psychological distress are five times higher, and some 30 percent of deaths in jails are due to suicide. Twenty percent of those incarcerated spend time in solitary confinement in a given year, which exacerbates the incidence of self-harm and violence.[21] All of this is worsened by unhealthy living conditions, including poor-quality food and housing, lack of adequate exercise, and tense environments.

At the same time, prisoners often lack access to needed treatment. "It's ironic that custodial environments are the only places where there's a constitutional right to health care in the United States," said Parsons, "yet those are the places where the health care is the worst." For example, people very rarely receive treatment for substance use disorders while incarcerated.

Health in the Family and in the Community

The social determinants of health model offers a framework for thinking about mass incarceration; involvement in the criminal justice system often undermines access to housing, employment, and education and interrupts Medicaid coverage and psychiatric care. Other family members, especially children, also feel the impact. "We have a simplistic view of the damages caused by incarceration and its costs because we're missing many of the more complex health impacts," said Parsons.

Areas in which a high percentage of residents are incarcerated tend to have high rates of diabetes, infant mortality, premature mortality, and psychiatric hospitalizations.[22] Overall, there is a 2.9 percent increase in community-wide morbidity in those communities.[23]

At the same time, almost all incarcerated people (95%) eventually return to their communities, bringing their health issues with them. Better care, both while incarcerated and after release, "will benefit the most unhealthy and vulnerable neighborhoods," said Parsons. "We need to do a better job with this population, both for justice system purposes and also for public health."

> *Within the health profession there is a lack of understanding of the impact of mass incarceration. Bringing it to the attention of public health professionals through use of social determinants of health and public health measures is really important.* —Jim Parsons

Interventions that Disrupt the Incarceration Cycle

The cycling of individuals through the criminal justice system, back to the community, and through the system once again can seem relentless, pulling ever more people and their families and communities into a vortex of poverty, ill health, and despair.

But local efforts to break the cycle offer hope. The four examples below tackle incarceration from different angles: the design of incarcerated environments, the involvement with the criminal justice system that threads through multiple generations, the lack of stable housing and social services that results in jail time for petty offenses, and minor drug-related misdemeanors that fill jails with low-threat sellers and users.

Transforming Conditions of Confinement

Restoring Promise, a Vera Institute of Justice initiative, works with prisons and jails to redesign these environments so "they become places which put human dignity at the core and prepare people for reentry by not dehumanizing them while incarcerated," said Parsons.[24,25]

In 2017, with assistance from Vera, the Connecticut Department of Corrections launched the T.R.U.E. program (truthfulness, respectfulness, understanding, and elevating) for men ages 18 to 25 at its Cheshire Correctional Institution. In the T.R.U.E. unit, the men are out of their cells all day, have access to programming and incentives that promote positive behavior, and are encouraged to develop relationships with correctional staff. Men serving life sentences act as their mentors.

Results have been striking: no acts of violence occurred in the first 18 months; recidivism has declined; solitary confinement is no longer in use; and the incarcerated men report feeling safer and more prepared to succeed, connected to family, and fairly treated. Corrections officers have reported that, "for the first time in their careers, they actually enjoy going to work," said Parsons. In March 2019, the TV news program *60 Minutes* reported on the experience of the incarcerated men, corrections officers, and wardens who participate in the T.R.U.E. program.[26]

Based on this success, Connecticut is expanding its program, and Massachusetts and South Carolina are signing on to develop programs as well.

> *We need examples of how corrections environments can be different. We have an idea of prisons or jails as very punitive and unhealthy places and there is no reason they have to be that way. —Jim Parsons*

Helping Parents and Their Children Break the Cycle

Just over half of the people in prison or jail are parents of children under the age of 18.[27] This represents 2.7 million U.S. children—one in 28. More than one in nine black children has a parent in prison or jail. A conservative estimate puts the number of children who have had a parent incarcerated at some point during childhood at 5.1 million.[28]

Incarceration is very much a family issue and a community issue—and we need to address both. —Teresa Eckrich Sommer

Sommer's work with colleagues Lindsay Chase-Lansdale and Terri Sabol at Northwestern University's Two-Generation Research Initiative that is based in family systems theory focuses on interventions designed to foster healthy childhood development and to help adults improve their education, career, and income. This two-generation approach holds particular promise for families living with incarceration, and especially for keeping both parents and their children out of the criminal justice system.

Early two-generation efforts tended to involve "light touch referrals" to a child care or high school general equivalency diploma (GED) program. Today, the evolved 2.0 version emphasizes high-quality early childhood education combined with a well-thought-out focus on parental career development and family-supporting wages. Sommer described two programs that take different paths towards these goals.

Educating Both Children and Parents Through CareerAdvance˚

Career*Advance˚*, a program operated by the Community Action Project of Tulsa County, Okla. (CAP Tulsa, which serves young children in low-income families), offers parents of children in early childhood education centers tuition-free courses at local community colleges. It also partners with elementary schools, adult basic education and GED programs, English language learner programs, employers, and others. Among the keys to its success:

- Parents attend community college in cohorts of 15, allowing them to support and learn from one another and ease the transition to college coursework.
- Parents receive cash incentives and supports, such as child care and parent-sensitive scheduling, which remove barriers to participation. They also receive coaching on navigating their college experience while parenting young children.
- Coursework is directed at the health care sector, where demand for workers is high, to prepare parents for a viable job.
- "Stackable training" allows students to learn, get a job, and return for further training. For example, a student could become a certified nursing assistant, then a licensed practical nurse, and finally a registered nurse, moving in and out of formal education while working and raising young children.

Sommer and colleagues are conducting a longitudinal study of parents of children receiving Head Start services that compares 150 parents involved with

Career*Advance*° with 137 parents not involved with Career*Advance*°.[29] The study parents are almost all mothers, and about a third are single parents. Their average age is 29, with average annual household income (family of four) just over $15,000. The group is ethnically and racially diverse (40% black, 28% white, 9% Hispanic, and 23% other, including Native American). About half have a high school degree or less and about half have tried to get some certification with varying levels of success. On average, their children are 4 years old.

Parental results after one year were encouraging:[30]

- Sixty-one percent of participants earned career certificates, compared with only 4 percent of the comparison group.
- Some 51 percent of participants found employment in the health care sector, compared with 27 percent of the comparison group.
- Parental income did not decline because incentive payments made up for decreased earnings, allowing participants to shift to part-time work that accommodated school schedules.
- Career*Advance*° participants were more successful at achieving certification and gaining employment in the health sector than were participants of other career pathway training programs.
- Parents' psychological well-being exceeded that of the comparison group. They demonstrated significantly more career commitment, self-efficacy, and optimism, and did not exhibit more stress or psychological distress, a possible concern when combining work, school, and the care of young children.

Researchers also considered the impact of the program on the children enrolled in Head Start.

- There was a small effect on overall attendance at Head Start, with children of Career*Advance*° parents attending about five more days per semester than children of the matched comparison group. Parents' participation in Career*Advance*° also had a significant positive impact on chronic absenteeism (missing 10% of Head Start days in a semester). Some 37 percent of children of parents in the program were chronically absent, compared with 59 percent of children in the comparison group.[31]
- The children in CAP Tulsa's Head Start program already were performing well above the national average in math skills, literacy, and inhibitory control. These benefits were maintained when the Career*Advance*° program was added to family life.[32]
- The biggest gains were found among children whose parents were the most ready for college (higher educational level, age, and income) and among children who were themselves the least ready for school.[33]

Thus, concluded Sommer, "adding a workforce training program for parents doesn't interfere with—and in some cases exceeds—the benefits children gain from high-quality early education."

Supporting the Development of Young Parents and Their Children

Founded in 1999, UTEC (formerly United Teen Equality Center) in Lawrence and Lowell, Mass., provides intensive coaching and workforce services to young adults, ages 17 to 25, who have been involved with the criminal justice system and often with gangs.

In fiscal year 2018, UTEC's programs touched more than 600 young people, with 148 enrolled in its full-time program model. Some 36 percent of the youth served are current or expectant parents. "These parents are trying to figure out their own development and how to master the world, and they're also trying to attend to the needs of very young children," said Sommer.

When incarcerated young parents are released, one of the biggest barriers they face in trying to return to work or school is how to care for their children. In 2017, UTEC launched its family-focused two-generation program, offering coordinated programming for both children and parents, to help these young people take control of their lives. A UTEC-operated early childhood education center provides a child-centered, social–emotional learning-based curriculum called Preschool PATHS®.[34]

At the same time, parents, who are mostly fathers, receive a related, parent-centered curriculum, Power PATH, along with paid job training in mattress recycling, woodworking, or food services. Coaches link them with supports, such as mental health and substance use disorder counseling, and time is devoted to discussing their roles as fathers, providers, and partners. On-site education prepares participants for a high school equivalency credential, and college credits are available for courses completed at UTEC.

> UTEC is an incredibly visionary leader with a proven track record with criminal and gang-involved youth. —Teresa Eckrich Sommer

With support from the Robert Wood Johnson Foundation (RWJF), Sommer and her colleagues entered into a research partnership with UTEC to study the evolving program and strengthen its design over time. An effectiveness study will follow if the program "gets big enough and well-received enough," said Sommer.

UTEC is the first organization to use the two-generation curricula (Preschool PATHS® for children and Power PATH for parents) to serve families in which a parent has been incarcerated. Beginning in September 2019, children and parents are working on developing the same core competencies in areas such as social–emotional development, cognitive development, academic achievement, and physical health and well-being. "What they're doing for both generations is remarkably aligned," Sommer noted. Before adding the early education center and two-generation programming, the overall UTEC program had shown positive results: recidivism among participants was about 15 percent, compared with a Massachusetts average of 50 percent. The newly added elements are likely to improve further the well-being of parents and children alike.

Out of Jail and Into Supportive Housing

In Denver, where housing prices are increasing faster than the national average and the housing supply is limited, large numbers of residents face chronic homelessness—a situation that can increase the risk of jail stays. Almost all (98%) of those experiencing chronic homelessness in the Denver metro area in 2018 were single men.[35]

The Urban Institute's Devlin Hanson described how homeless people can rotate through the criminal justice system. "A homeless person sleeping on a park bench would receive a noncustodial arrest (citation and court date) from a police officer. The individual would not show up for the court date, an arrest warrant would be issued, and the next interaction with police would lead to jail. After time in jail, this person would be back on the street, still homeless and still looking for a place to sleep. The cycle would continue as the individual committed nuisance offenses like panhandling and trespassing."

Permanent housing, accompanied by a range of supportive services, is a promising solution to a costly problem. Studies find that as many as 80 percent of people who have been chronically homeless remain housed one year later, are significantly less likely to use shelters, and spend fewer days in jail.[36]

Housing the Homeless Through Social Impact Bond Financing

Lacking a clear funding source, the need for supportive housing to break the cycle of homelessness and incarceration is a candidate for social impact bond financing. An innovative way to tackle stubborn social concerns, social impact bond financing allows private investors to fund programs and assume risk. If a program works, the government pays back the funders with interest ("pay for success"); if not, the investors bear the loss.

Eight private investors (philanthropies and banks) and the City and County of Denver launched the Denver Supportive Housing Social Impact Bond Initiative in January 2016. In one of the country's first such efforts, the private investors provided $8.6 million in upfront capital for services, and the project leveraged additional state and local resources for permanent housing subsidies. Outcome measures have been established and will be rigorously evaluated.

A mix of other partners is key to this endeavor. The Colorado Coalition for the Homeless and the Mental Health Center of Denver provide the services while the Corporation for Supportive Housing and Enterprise Community Partners manage the initiative. Under a contract with the City of Denver, the Urban Institute, the Evaluation Center at University of Colorado, Denver, and the Burns Center on Poverty and Homelessness are conducting a randomized controlled trial to evaluate the impacts of supportive housing on housing stability and jail stays. With support from RWJF, the Urban Institute and partners also are evaluating the effects of the program on health services utilization.

The Denver Supportive Housing Model

The model is "housing first" with low barriers to entry—an individual does not have to be sober, for example, to be accepted. Residents are provided services intended to keep them stably housed, including behavioral health and substance use disorder treatment; food resources; legal referrals; and medical, dental, and vision care.

Using criminal justice data, project partners identified and referred 363 individuals to supportive housing in the project's first two years. Most were men (84%) in their forties and fifties, with an average of 14 arrests, of which seven were noncustodial, or ticket, arrests. The group was 40 percent white, 33 percent black, 18 percent Hispanic, and 8 percent Native American. Many had been on the street for more than three years and had multiple health and substance use challenges. Based on data from homeless services providers, this population did not spend much time in emergency shelters and typically faced many barriers to consistent health care.

Provider partners had to modify their usual intake process for this highly vulnerable population, which was not actively seeking services. The referral pathway designed to target these individuals required a different outreach process because they could be located only by a name and last known contact. Despite concerns about the feasibility of the process, providers found 86 percent of the first 363 individuals referred to supportive housing. Of those, 90 percent agreed to accept housing, and 86 percent of that group received housing vouchers. Of those with vouchers, 96 percent signed leases. The total process from referral to signed lease took an average of 57 days.

That process came with many challenges. Because of previous trauma and barriers to services, people were very fearful about engaging, and building trust and finding key documents (such as birth certificates and Social Security cards) required substantial effort. Bridge housing proved to be a real boon, giving individuals a safe place to stay and allowing providers to find them as their applications were processed.

"This is a huge life transition for these individuals," stressed Hanson. Living on the street for so long, they were reluctant to leave their social networks behind. An outreach behavioral health navigator helped them adjust to housing and to the "scary steps along the way."

Interim Results: Staying Housed

The five-year evaluation includes a process study of program implementation and a randomized controlled impact study. Of the 285 participants housed from the program's inception in January 2016 through June 2018:

- Some 85 percent remained housed without ever having exited the program.
- Some 44 percent had no jail stays after one year in housing, and most of the others had been jailed only once.[37] The overall average number of days in jail for the housed population during that year was 19, compared with the average of 77 days in a year typical for this population prior to program entry.

The research team considers these results encouraging, but the true impacts of the study will be revealed by the future results of the randomized controlled trial. The team emphasizes the importance of daily, custom-tailored support from service providers, as well as the collaboration with police and health care providers that is also critical to housing stability.

"The program is showing early promise, but there's a lot of work ahead," said Hanson. The impact study will address the question of whether supportive housing decreases use of costly public services, with results expected in May 2021.

Treatment, Not Arrest, for People With Substance Use Disorders

Chicago is a major hub of heroin use and distribution, yet Chicago police officers "take pride when they can avoid incarcerating someone they don't believe is a danger to public safety," said Harold Pollack of the University of Chicago. Although people with substance use disorders—low-level street dealers and their buyers—are the easiest offenders to arrest, police prefer to get them off the street and into treatment.

An Arrest Alternative

The Westside Narcotics Diversion and Treatment Initiative, launched in March 2016, is a collaboration of the Chicago Police Department, University of Chicago Urban Labs, and the High Intensity Drug Trafficking Areas Program (which co-ordinates local, state, and federal drug-control efforts). Supported by RWJF, the pilot program involved three treatment providers: Haymarket Center, Heartland Health Outreach, and Thresholds.

> *Our law enforcement partners really were enthusiastic to do this. They were desperate to find some way to help people with substance use disorders consistent with public safety.* —Harold Pollack

Pollack described the approach as more about "deflection" than diversion. Formal diversion programs generally target those who need intense monitoring and supervision, with sanctions imposed for transgressions. Deflection is entirely voluntary and aims to keep an individual out of the system altogether. Generally, it is a one-shot opportunity—if the police keep encountering an individual, that person becomes ineligible for it. "For someone who is not a threat to public safety, deflection is often a very good way to help," said Pollack.

For the pilot, police officers detained people who purchased heroin from undercover officers in a "reverse sting." They were screened for eligibility: in possession of one gram or less of a controlled substance, having a substance use disorder, and being willing to accept treatment. Program disqualifiers included being on parole or probation, an arrest warrant, conviction for a violent crime, gang involvement, or being viewed by police as a public safety threat. Police took those eligible to a treatment facility for intake; anyone who refused intake would be arrested and charged with a misdemeanor.

Pollack and his colleagues studied 39 deflection-eligible individuals detained in the reverse sting. Their average age was 47 and they were mostly male (87%) and predominantly black (69%); the remainder were white (21%) and Hispanic or "other" (10%). Almost all (37 of 39) had an arrest history, with a total of 320 arrests, mostly related to drugs. They had not been criminally active immediately prior to detainment.

Participants spent an average of 2.2 inpatient and 21.7 outpatient days in treatment—less than an optimal length of time, noted Pollack. The hope is that treatment will reduce their level of drug use, but as Pollack said, "these are people that may have been using heroin for 25, 30, 40 years in some cases. This is not their first rodeo. It would be better if we could improve retention, but recovery is a long process with lots of bumps in the road and this is a particularly intensive population."

Pilot Results

After eight months in the program, re-offending rates were low: three people had been arrested, two for minor issues and one for a domestic violence felony.

"I am convinced that most of the people served can be safely deflected to treatment because they are not public safety threats in the first place," said Pollack. Though some were homeless or unemployed, many were older working-class Chicagoans, often African Americans, with long-standing heroin use disorders. When the sting took place at 7:30 in the morning, some were headed to blue-collar jobs. "There's no reason for the criminal justice system to interact with them in a coercive way."

Pollack highlighted two factors that he regards as distinctive about this program: the high degree of law enforcement buy-in and the flexibility of providers. Referral to treatment through deflection, although voluntary, is random and abrupt. People are not presenting themselves after making a conscious decision to seek treatment nor are they under a court order to do so. Providers must focus on harm reduction as they try to persuade people to accept treatment, rather than insist on complete withdrawal.

Sharing the Benefits

Encouraged by the pilot results, the Chicago Police Department is putting the procedures of the Westside program into everyday policing practice. A clinician from Thresholds, one of the pilot providers, performs screening and assessments on-site at the police department daily. "A common thing you'll hear from police leaders is that we cannot arrest our way out of our crime problem," said Pollack.

Faith in Indiana: Changing the Narrative

Remember when everyone was mad at Reagan because he was throwing everybody in jail and then Clinton got in and threw more people in jail? It doesn't matter about the regime if the narrative hasn't changed. —Juard Barnes

Faith in Indiana is a diverse coalition of people from 17 faith traditions acting together for racial and economic justice. It is part of the national Faith in Action network, which seeks transformation through action on economic dignity, gun violence, health care, immigrant justice, mass incarceration, and voting rights. The vision of Faith in Indiana, said Juard Barnes, former deputy director and now at Faith in Action, is that "people of faith can come together in a region and affect change socially and politically."

The coalition believes passionately that racial attitudes and actions are woven into the nation's fabric, and that the narratives on incarceration, immigration, and race must be changed. Barnes cited the racialization of crime and poverty, and the portrayal of immigrants as "rapists and murderers," as examples of narratives that hold people back. The coalition's framing includes these themes:

- People have the power to transform a region; jobs are needed, not jails.
- When people are treated with dignity and have opportunities, they don't rob.
- Most people in the black community and the poor white community are not looking for anybody to kill. They're looking for someplace to work and to take care of their families.
- We all are family and we all speak to the human, to the circle of dignity. America can stand powerfully united across race, gender, and ideology in a way that doesn't compromise anyone.
- Powerful ways can be found to truly communicate at a grassroots level.

The work is "steeped in the stories of our people," said Barnes, stories that speak to a system of oppression as the "real culprit," where the telling often begins: "I was raised in poverty and we didn't have food in our house and I got caught up trying to find money for food." Or: "My father was in jail and he was gone."

The Power of Public Action

Faith in Indiana organizes public events to call attention to a policy, program, or issue it wants to influence. A strategy team works on tactics, a clergy council clarifies the theological basis for the work, toolkits teach people how to hold house meetings, and a captain guides the process. "Buckets" are created for media, logistics, turnout, and agenda.

In a "research action," a small team meets with key civic or political leaders whose support is critical—typically, a mayor, governor, or another official—to share evidence about an issue. To ensure a leader's support, said Barnes, "the single, most powerful thing is a research action."

Once the official offers support, the group agrees on questions to be asked at a public event, with the media present. Members recruit a crowd to attend, and the targeted official states his or her public agreement. In Indiana, these public actions are changing the narrative on poverty, crime, and incarceration.

A Smaller, Beefier Criminal Justice Center

The Faith in Indiana approach had one of its major successes in Marion County. When the new Criminal Justice Center opens in 2022, it will include a county jail with 3,000 beds, along with a county courthouse. It also will include an assessment and intervention center providing mentally ill offenders (30% to 40% of those involved with the county criminal justice system) with wraparound services to "stop the revolving door of justice," said Indianapolis mayor Joe Hogsett at the groundbreaking.[38] "What we seek is a criminal justice system that saves more lives than it detains."

That was not always the plan. The original design for the center was a 4,000-bed jail (1,500 beds more than the existing facility) with no mental health services and no criminal justice reforms. But activists from Faith in Indiana knew that the absence of mental health resources was a big factor in incarceration. A poor pretrial process and problems with the bail system also were keeping people in jail longer than necessary.

"We began a fight," Barnes admitted.

Faith in Indiana members surveyed 10,000 people about the plan, and some 86 percent agreed that a better strategy was needed. The coalition then conducted "research actions" with 22 of the 29 city councilors, explaining what they had learned from other U.S. cities: if police are trained, mental health and drug treatment services are available, drug courts and employment programs are in place, and the bail system is reformed, then "people won't have to be sitting in jail."

The fight went on for a year. Eventually, the coalition persuaded several councilors to stand publicly with them, the city council voted against the old plan, the mayor did not run for another term, and the new mayor agreed to adopt the new plan, reducing the bed size of the new jail and incorporating the reforms for which Faith in Indiana had advocated. In addition, the Indiana Supreme Court voted to end cash bail as of January 2018.

In a related effort, the Mobile Crisis Alert Team (MCAT) launched in August 2017. MCAT deploys a patrol officer, a paramedic, and a licensed mental health clinician to emergency calls involving mental health or addiction issues. After five months, an evaluation by the Indiana Public Policy Institute found that only 2 percent of the people with whom MCAT intervened went to jail.[39] Two-thirds of the time, the patrol officer was able to depart, leaving other team members to handle the case.

> *This was a powerful movement, and it's changed the whole face of our city. Now when people talk about criminal justice in Indianapolis, the narrative has changed. They talk about mental health, about jobs, and about bail instead of about these bad people who need to be put in jail.* —Juard Barnes

A Final Word

The causes and effects of mass incarceration in the United States are complex, and effective solutions to this crisis of equity, health, and well-being for individuals, families, and communities will not be easily implemented. Still, there is hope as parties across the political spectrum increasingly acknowledge the critical need for reform.

The bipartisan legislation enacted by Congress in December 2018 will likely improve functioning and outcomes within the federal prison system. Elsewhere, new ideas are being developed and tested to prevent incarceration, improve conditions and treatment for those who are incarcerated, and assist people released from jail and prison in reconnecting with their families and communities.

As a social determinant of health, incarceration is especially layered and complicated. Being or having been incarcerated has wide-ranging physical, mental, social, and economic health consequences. Incarceration also can limit access to other determinants, such as housing and employment. But viewed from another angle, the incarcerated setting offers opportunities to recognize the humanity and dignity of those it houses and to provide quality services that prepare them for a more productive life upon release.

The work described in this chapter addresses multiple points along the incarceration continuum that can change both the narrative and the reality of incarceration. Examining the many impacts of mass incarceration as a social justice issue, including as a significant barrier to racial equity, can help break the cycle and develop more supportive care systems and healthier people, families, and communities.

Chapter 6 Spotlight: Fathers Mentoring Fathers

Vance Simms, Founder/Executive Director, Father Matters

A package of chocolate chip cookies, a pot of coffee, and four kitchen chairs in a studio apartment in San Jose, Calif., set the stage for the inaugural meeting in 1997 of what would evolve into Father Matters. Now located in Phoenix and built on the idea of fathers mentoring fathers, Father Matters provides support to fathers as young as 15 and to mothers as well, serving about 3,800 people each year.

Executive Director Vance Simms founded Father Matters when, as a 22-year-old unmarried father, he battled his son's mother on custody issues. Attending court-ordered parenting courses, he became committed to the idea of bringing together men, of any race or background, "who just want to be great dads to their children."

For seven years Simms worked full-time driving a Frito Lay potato chip truck while using his own money to run evening and weekend workshops and support groups. As the groups expanded, Simms self-published Dear Nathan: A Young Man's Journey to Fatherhood, *a memoir written as a letter to his son, and began offering his mentoring program to court systems, churches, and social service agencies. In time, these efforts coalesced into the structured organization it is today.*[1]

Simms believes that absent fathers foster anger in their children that can result in gang involvement, drug abuse, and other reactions to mask the pain. "Men are growing up very angry at their fathers," said Simms.

The premise of Father Matters is about "taking people from where they are to where they want to be. I can't do anything about what you did 11 years ago, that got you nine years, and now you can't get credit, can't find a place to rent, your family moved to a different state because they're embarrassed about what you did." The program starts right there, mostly with self-referrals that typically come through word of mouth or Facebook.

At Father Matters, an individual cannot show up on Thursday morning and expect staff to "pull all these rabbits out of the hat" to help them deal with a court date the following Monday. "I don't allow people to waste our time," Simms stressed, "but I also don't allow us to waste their time."

Customers, as they are called, first go through an intake process to identify their service needs. When they return, the caseworker is prepared with a package of needed supports: bus cards, food vouchers, and phone numbers for other resources. At the next appointment, the customer is expected to have completed a set of assignments. "It's called following through," said Simms. "When you come to Father Matters, you better be ready to make a life change."

Almost 30 percent of participating fathers have been incarcerated. Father Matters also works with men who will be released shortly from prison to help them develop plans for life on the outside. To ensure the feasibility of these plans, the organization connects with the men's families as well.

People coming out of prison or jail typically need housing and a job first, said Simms, along with life skills. Their communities are likely to have changed, and Father Matters helps them reconnect. Many start by volunteering at the organization—an opportunity to gain experience and receive a letter of support they can use with employers who are familiar with the organization. "These employers know when they're getting someone from Father Matters, they're getting a soldier."

Within support groups, men who have been in prison, and those who have not, learn from one another. "Men don't know how to speak to each other. We're always in competition," said Simms. "We break all that down because, in the end, most of us are still dealing with little-boy issues: insecurity, low self-esteem, worry." The staff strives to get under these issues and help fathers move forward.

In addition to parenting classes, support groups, and one-on-one counseling sessions, Father Matters offers legal assistance, resource referrals, help in applying for public benefits, supervised visits with children, monitored exchanges of children between parents to avoid conflict, and a range of workshops.

"Tiny details can make the difference," Simms has learned. Bus cards allow people to get to support groups and workshops, then to interviews, and finally to jobs, all before the first paycheck has arrived. Father Matters also provides appropriate clothes for interviews and work and freely dispenses advice, such as to scope out interview locations in order to estimate travel time, to arrive early, and to dress the part. "You have to do life with them," he said, reciting the Father Matters mantra. People are generally connected with the organization for six months to a year.

Relationships with providers in social services and criminal justice circles have helped it grow. Phoenix probation officers see almost 200 people each week on-site at Father Matters, and probationers can then receive other needed services. Simms speaks to many organizations and hosts a weekly radio program; in addition, the bimonthly Father Matters Tribune has over 7,000 subscribers. Grants, speaking engagements, federal contracts, and proceeds from the sale of Simms's three books provide funding.

"People know when you come to Father Matters it's like coming to my living room, kicking it on the couch with a cold root beer, talking about the day," said Simms. Ultimately it comes down to leading people to "forgiveness," and "listening to people with the heart, treating them with respect, and following through."

The Opioid Epidemic

Busting Myths and Sharing Solutions

James Becker, MD, Medicaid Medical Director, West Virginia Department of Health and Human Resources

Brendan Saloner, PhD, Assistant Professor, Johns Hopkins Bloomberg School of Public Health

Joshua M. Sharfstein, MD, Professor of the Practice in Health Policy and Management, Johns Hopkins Bloomberg School of Public Health

Jeffery Talbert, PhD, Professor, Department of Pharmacy Practice and Science, University of Kentucky

R. Corey Waller, MD, Health Management Associates, Emergency Medicine and Addiction specialist

When life expectancy in the United States declined for the third year in a row in 2017, a sobering array of statistics pointed to one irrefutable factor to help explain the longest sustained life expectancy decline in more than a century: the nation's escalating opioid epidemic.

In 2017, over 70,000 people in this country died from drug overdoses, up from a record high of nearly 64,000 in 2106. For perspective, this exceeds the number of people killed in a year from motor vehicle accidents, which have historically been the nation's leading cause of death. It also exceeds the death rate at the height of the HIV/AIDS epidemic in the early 1990s.[1] This death-by-overdose epidemic, experts agree, represents a public health crisis of unprecedented proportions.

In this chapter, five researchers and physicians discuss the opioid epidemic, address the myths that surround it, and identify possible solutions. Joshua M. Sharfstein offers an overview on the extent and nature of the nationwide crisis, while Brendan Saloner presents grim statistics, reviews immediate steps that can make a difference, and details a new treatment approach in Delaware.

Culture of Health in Practice, Alonzo L. Plough. Oxford University Press (2020) © Robert Wood Johnson Foundation
DOI: 10.1093/oso/9780190071400.001.0001

James Becker provides a physician's unvarnished description of treating overdose victims in West Virginia, and Jeffery Talbert focuses the lens on Kentucky,
with both sections serving as a reminder that "place matters" in this epidemic.
R. Corey Waller, an addiction and emergency medicine specialist, describes the
public health crisis as a crisis of addiction and not one of opioids only. Finally,
in a Spotlight on rural addiction, Becker borrows from his lived experiences in
West Virginia to help explain why this is such a devastating problem in rural
America.

"So Staggering": The Opioid Epidemic in Numbers

> Myth: Publicity about the opioid epidemic has helped eliminate the
> problem.
> Fact: The high level of recognition about the opioid crisis has not stopped it.

Joshua M. Sharfstein of the Johns Hopkins Bloomberg School of Public Health
readily acknowledged a tragic conundrum. Despite considerable publicity about
the country's worst-ever drug epidemic, overdose deaths from opioids are on
the rise. The nation has looked repeatedly at stories and photos of people with
addictions injecting others in abandoned houses; at online videos of overdosed
adults passed out on the sidewalk, their children still strapped in car seats
nearby; at documentaries of emergency medical services (EMS) crews working
frantically to save the life of an overdose victim. And yet the number of deaths
keep growing.

> The high level of recognition about the opioid epidemic has not stopped
> the crisis. We have so far not been able to turn the corner on a very serious
> problem. —Joshua M. Sharfstein

When the Centers for Disease Control and Prevention (CDC) released the
most recent opioid epidemic statistics in November 2018,[2] Sharfstein's definitive response to those numbers became a national headline in the *New York
Times*: "The numbers are so staggering."[3]
  According to the CDC:

- Some 70,237 drug overdose deaths occurred in the United States in 2017,
  compared with 63,632 in 2016. Nonprescription opioids such as fentanyl and
  heroin were involved in 47,600 of these deaths, that is, in more than two-
  thirds of them.

- Overdose death rates increased for both men and women, with the highest rates among adults ages 25 to 44. In 2017, the per capita overdose death rate in the United States (21.7 per 100,000) was nearly 10 percent higher than the rate in 2016 (19.8 per 100,000).
- The steep increase over the last three years contributed to a shortened life expectancy in the United States. In a pattern not seen since World War I and the flu pandemic in the early 20th century, life expectancy at birth fell by nearly four months to 78.6 years. (Early indicators of this trend were described by Anne Case and Angus Deaton at the 2016 *Sharing Knowledge* conference, and are included in Volume 1 of this series;[4] they also were published in the *Proceedings of the National Academy of Sciences*.[5]) Although suicide, other forms of violence, and an increase in chronic illnesses such as obesity also play a role in this decline, "The rapid change in death rates over the last few years makes the opioid epidemic stand out," said Sharfstein. "Life expectancy is improving in many places in the world. It shouldn't be decreasing in the United States."

It's important to note that these numbers focus only on overdose deaths. The overall scope of the problem is even worse. In 2017, approximately 7.5 million people had some kind of a drug-use disorder (excluding alcohol-related disorders); an estimated 2.1 million of them identified as having an opioid use disorder, through prescription or street drugs.[6]

"America has struggled with opioids since the Civil War," said Sharfstein, who leads the Bloomberg American Health Initiative at Johns Hopkins. "What makes today's epidemic so extraordinary is the scale of overdose deaths. We have an incredibly serious problem."

Changing Patterns, Disproportionate Impact

Myth: Prescription opioids are driving a worsening opioid epidemic.
Fact: Although opioid prescription rates remain a critical problem in rural areas, the use of prescription opioids is actually decreasing in many regions.

Brendan Saloner, Sharfstein's Johns Hopkins colleague at the Bloomberg School of Public Health and co-lead of the addiction and overdose track at the Bloomberg American Health Initiative, did not mince words in remarking, "I think it's fair to say this is a public health crisis of unprecedented proportions." Saloner emphasized several important facts about substance use disorders and opioids.

First, patterns of use are changing, which helps to dispel the myth that pre-scription drugs remain the primary driver of the epidemic. Deaths involving syn-thetic, nonprescription opioids such as fentanyl and fentanyl analogs increased more than 45 percent in 2017 alone,[7] while overdose death rates involving nat-ural and semisynthetic opioids (oxycodone and hydrocodone), heroin, and methadone remained unchanged. "Fentanyl really seems to be one of the main reasons why the overdose numbers continued to surge so much in the last couple years," Saloner explained.

Synthetic opioid drugs tend to be deadlier than prescription drugs because they are more potent; even a small error in measurement can trigger an over-dose. And the mere fact that these drugs keep evolving—which threatens to make responses obsolete before they can even get started—is one of the factors that makes the opioid problem so unique, explained James Becker of the West Virginia Department of Health and Human Resources.

"In our community of Huntington, we started out in the 1990s with people abusing a prescription drug like oxycodone primarily, or morphine," said Becker, laying out the timeline for one community's ever-evolving drug habits. "Then, as the supply of that medication got expensive, and we put controls in place for prescriptions, people switched over to the less expensive drugs like heroin."

Heroin was dominant in Huntington for five to 10 years, until cheap syn-thetic opiates began coming in from China. Then, as word spread about their dangers, people again changed their patterns, adding inexpensive supplies of methamphetamine to the mix. "So today, on the streets in Huntington," Becker explained, "if you bought drugs from somebody, you would probably be buying a combination of some fentanyl and meth and that's a different scenario than where we were with heroin five years ago."

Second, prescription opioid use is actually decreasing. According to the CDC, the total number of prescriptions peaked in 2012 at 81.3 prescriptions per 100 persons; by 2017 that rate had fallen to its lowest in more than 10 years, at 58.7 prescriptions per 100 persons.[8] Nonetheless, rates in the United States still far exceed its peer countries.

Third, "This is a crisis that has had disproportionate impact on certain communities," stressed Saloner. Although whites are disproportionately affected in many areas, overdoses are rising most rapidly among African Americans in eastern cities[9] and increasingly impacting Native American communities as well. And the opioid epidemic has had a particularly acute impact on rural communities.

Rural Communities Grapple With Opioids

Drug use in rural communities was at the forefront of a 2018 "Life in Rural America" survey conducted for National Public Radio, the Robert Wood Johnson Foundation, and the Harvard T. H. Chan School of Public Health.[10]

> *Rural Americans identify drug addiction . . . and economic concerns as the two biggest problems facing their local communities. In particular, opioid addiction/abuse have had major impacts on the lives of rural Americans. —* "Life in Rural America" report

The survey found that a majority of rural residents agree that opioid addiction is a serious problem in their community, and almost one-quarter identify addiction as the most urgent health problem currently facing their community. Nearly half the survey respondents say the problem has gotten worse over the past five years, and half have personally known someone who has struggled with opioid addiction.[11] (A rural physician gives his personal perspective on the depth of rural America's struggle with the opioid epidemic in "Spotlight: Rural Addiction: A Perfect Storm, a Nod to Grandma, Pills for Cash.")

According to the CDC, the highest rates of death due to drug overdose in 2017 were in West Virginia (57.8 per 100,000), Ohio (46.3 per 100,000), Pennsylvania (44.3 per 100,000), the District of Columbia (44.0 per 100,000), and Kentucky (37.2 per 100,000).

While the high overdose rate in Washington, DC, reflects fentanyl's steady growth in U.S. cities, the state statistics illustrate how rural communities have been affected. A recent study supported by the Bloomberg American Health Initiative highlighted the opioid epidemic in West Virginia; according to the report, 20 percent of the state's overdoses were in just one county, Cabell County, which is 80 percent rural.[12] (See Chapter 3, "Pathways to Change in Rural America," for more about the unique vulnerabilities—and special strengths—of rural areas that help fuel the opioid epidemic and perhaps offer ways out of it.)

Despite the overall decline in prescription rates, the connection between opioid prescribing and overdose deaths in rural communities is stark, as two maps of Kentucky illustrate. The University of Kentucky's Jeffery Talbert drew a bright red circle on each map—one showing the parts of the state with the highest opioid prescribing rates, the other showing the highest overdose death rates. The red circles were in *exactly* the same southeast corner of the state, and included three rural counties that rank among the country's 10 top-prescribing counties.

You see the same counties in the map of the rolling three-year average of
death from overdose and in the map of prescribing rates. So, again, it matters
where you live. —Jeffery Talbert

Bringing Statistics to Life: Images of Addiction

Myth: The opioid epidemic is an addiction problem, and people addicted to
opioids are all the same.

Fact: The opioid epidemic is a medical, mental health, behavioral, and soci-
etal problem. The population addicted to opioids is not homogenous, which
complicates treatment and other solutions.

People who struggle with addiction come from many backgrounds, "covering the full diversity of race, religion, economic group, and geography," said
Sharfstein. Many dwell in families and communities with the broad social and
environmental challenges that impede a Culture of Health. Indeed, measures of
community well-being—or their absence—help predict addiction, noted Carol
Graham, PhD, the Leo Pasvolsky Senior Fellow at the Brookings Institution.[13]
Poverty, intergenerational trauma, inadequate schools and health care, lack of
employment opportunities, and mental illness are all factors that can fuel despair.

These are really distressed families that have complex challenges that go
beyond the sort of biological symptoms of opioid use disorder. —Brendan
Saloner

The "dual challenge" of substance use disorder and untreated serious mental illness is a further burden. "These epidemics have a particularly daunting impact
on rural communities, where the rate of opioid-related overdose deaths is 45 percent higher than in metro-area counties," states "Communities in Crisis: Local
Responses to Behavioral Health Challenges," a 2017 report funded by the RWJF
and published by Manatt Health. "Smaller cities and counties have a lower tax
base and fewer resources . . . resulting in more limited access to care and treatment relative to urban centers."[14]

Calling the opioid epidemic "multifactorial," Becker pointed that it is "a medical problem and a mental health behavior problem, and a social ill that needs
addressing. And it's the convergence of these problems that has made this such
a difficult problem to address. The patients that we're trying to help, some have
mental illness. Some have horrible social situations like homelessness or a violent past. Some are victims of accidents. That lack of homogeneity is probably
the single greatest challenge in managing this kind of population."

Huntington, W.Va.: Scenes From the Epidemic

What does the opioid epidemic look like in a rural community in West Virginia? As both state medical director and a family practitioner in Cabell County, which includes rural communities in and around Huntington, W.Va., Becker is painfully familiar with scenes from that crisis.

From 2015 to 2017, West Virginia's overdose deaths grew from 41.5 to 57.8 deaths per 100,000, more than double the national average. Like Kentucky, West Virginia has among the highest number of painkiller prescriptions per person. "Our state is notorious for its reliance on pharmaceutical solutions, and we lead the country in reliance on prescription medication," said Becker.

Drug overdose deaths in the state have risen every year since 2017, when use of heroin, fentanyl, and carfentanil (a stronger version of fentanyl) started to spike. The opioid epidemic correlates with higher rates of some infectious diseases, especially HIV and hepatitis C virus (HCV) among people who inject drugs.

The epidemic also correlates to a dramatic increase in West Virginia's foster care cases and the presence of neonatal abstinence syndrome (NAS), a constellation of conditions that occur when babies withdraw from drugs they were exposed to in utero. "Eighty percent of those children in foster care have been taken out of homes where substance use disorder is an issue," Becker said. Between 2014 and 2016, 37 in 1,000 babies were born with NAS.

Becker has repeatedly witnessed these statistics playing out in everyday life. Although he described a few of his medical encounters in calm, measured terms, his vivid narrative was shocking:

> "I live in a community where 28 people overdosed in a three-hour period in one afternoon. Two of them were in the lobby of the medical center where I practice. One of them was deceased in the restroom, just outside our pharmacy. And I gave somebody Narcan in the lobby. So this is the kind of environment that we're in these days. . . .
>
> "I was interviewing and examining a 24-year-old woman, a heroin user, and I was surprised when I got to her gynecologic history that she had had no pregnancies. In fact, she said she had an IUD. It's fairly rare in our area to find someone who's using any form of contraception— one of the reasons we have this horrible NAS rate—so that's kind of remarkable. So I said to her, 'This [birth control] is a good decision on your part. You're coming in here to detox from heroin. You've made a good decision.' And her words to me were, 'No person should have to live their life trying to recover from their childhood.'"

Searching for Solutions

Myth: Treating opioid addiction doesn't work. Drug addiction should be a crime.

Fact: Treating opioid addiction does work. Drug addiction should not be a crime.

Many experts agree that some of the approaches to the opioid epidemic actually make the problem worse. They reviewed strategies that *don't* work, and then segued into the countervailing solutions more likely to turn the tide.

Harm Reduction

Keeping medical treatments from people with addiction makes the problem worse. Expanding the availability of harm reduction tools—such as medications for opioid use disorder, naloxone, syringe services, and fentanyl test strips—is a solution.

Saloner advocates "expanding the suite of harm reduction tools that we know are very effective." Harm reduction tools are a useful adjunct to three, FDA-approved drugs: methadone and buprenorphine, which help to reduce withdrawal symptoms, and naltrexone, which blocks people from experiencing the high normally associated with opioid use.[15]

For people experiencing the acute symptoms of an overdose, an injection of an opioid antagonist called naloxone (brand names Narcan° and Evzio°) quickly restores normal respiration. First responders and other medical professionals can inject naloxone, but it is also available in many pharmacies without a prescription and can be dispensed to family members of those who obtain prescription opioids for pain. In Virginia, for example, prescription opioid users are given a naloxone prescription simultaneously.

Talbert acknowledged some controversy about naloxone, referencing an ongoing debate over the "moral hazard" of naloxone, and whether its increased availability could actually worsen the problem by making opioids more appealing.[16] But Becker wasn't buying the argument, confirming his strong support of naloxone programs. Saloner agreed with Becker.

Medication works. Treatment works. So there can't be any controversy on that topic. If this is busting myths, we have to be just very, very clear about that. —Brendan Saloner

Two other harm reduction tools are fentanyl test strips (intended to help people understand what is in the drugs they purchased) and needle exchange programs that dispense sterile syringes and provide a place for drug users to discard their used needles. The exchange programs are designed, in part, to curb hepatitis C and HIV outbreaks, but equally importantly, they provide an opportunity to offer medical and counseling services.

The needle exchange programs have nonetheless become controversial, with opponents arguing that they normalize the use of deadly drugs. In April 2018, a program in Charleston, W.Va., closed after nearly two years of operation when it was overwhelmed by too many users and the health department struggled with complaints about discarded needles.[17]

But professionals in the field typically view needle exchange programs as essential resources, as well as an avenue for discussions about treatment and harm reduction. "The real benefit is not the exchange of the needle," said Becker. "The real benefit is the contact with somebody who potentially needs or wants recovery, and then getting to know that individual and getting them to know you really make a difference."

Emergency medicine physician Corey Waller, a strong proponent of needle exchange programs, argued that harm reduction *is* treatment. "When I'm in the emergency department and I give somebody a stack of needles out of the drawer because they need them, that's treatment. And if we have supervised injection sites, that's treatment. We're dealing more with the stigma and discrimination of the disease when people don't realize that that's treatment."

Barriers to Treatment

Putting up barriers to medical treatment makes the problem worse. Providing low-threshold treatment options is a solution.

"Low-threshold treatment" means eliminating barriers that would otherwise keep people from entering treatment programs. Some examples: Increasing treatment capacity to move people off waiting lists; not requiring full abstinence as a criterion for continuing care, and expanding the use of medications for opioid addiction treatment. "You just try to meet people where they're at and start them with treatment immediately," said Saloner. "It's not only a public health strategy, it's also a harm reduction strategy."

Treatment, Not Jail

Treating addiction as a criminal problem makes the problem worse. Reorienting criminal justice to divert from incarceration and provide treatment to people suffering from addiction advances solutions.

In various parts of the country, and through recent federal legislation, efforts to decriminalize drug use and erase the stigma of addiction have gained momentum.

In addition, many prosecutors across the country have announced that they will no longer prosecute marijuana possession misdemeanors. "Success will require rethinking the historic stigma and criminalization of people who use drugs illicitly," said Sharfstein.

The second step in this reform movement is rethinking how to treat opioid addiction behind bars. "There's very good evidence that arresting people, leaving them to withdraw from opioids, and sending them back out onto the streets raises the risk of overdose," said Sharfstein. "That's because people lose their tolerance while in detention and the same dose of opioids that they previously used may now be fatal."

(The links between substance use disorders and the criminal justice system, and the results of community-based interventions designed to break the cycle, are more fully described in Chapter 6, "Disrupting the Cycle of Incarceration.")

Saloner underscored the importance of reorienting how law enforcement officials respond to people with opioid use disorders. "There needs to be a real rethinking of how police interact with people in the wake of an overdose or with that person in the possession of opioids. Police should stop arresting people for being in possession of buprenorphine, which they will do if they think that the person doesn't legally have a prescription for that medication. That makes no sense from a public health perspective."

Waller took it one step further, arguing that "people should not be criminalized for having a disease. Period. And if that disease includes methamphetamine or cocaine or whatever, they shouldn't go to jail for that disease. They should be treated for that."

> *When you put criminal history into a medical record, that makes me angry. Because the minute you connect a medical decision to a criminal background check, you've now broken the oath that we have as physicians.* —Corey Waller

Glimmers of Hope

By late 2018, there were encouraging signs that 2017 could represent the peak of the opioid overdose epidemic. Preliminary CDC data showed that death rates from opioid drug overdose had leveled off nationally from January to August 2018, though the rate of deaths from synthetic opioids (excluding methadone) continued to increase.[18]

Though Sharfstein remained concerned—"the concept of a plateau doesn't fill me with a lot of optimism, given how high the numbers are," he told the *New York Times*—there are glimmers of hope in innovative programs across the country. By and large, these programs recognize the value of rapid access to effective medications and the importance of addressing stigma, adopting a "whole community" approach, and moving away from traditional criminal justice strategies:

- **In Rhode Island, a treatment program for opioid addiction launched by the state Department of Corrections in 2016 was associated with a significant drop in post-incarceration drug overdose deaths and contributed to an overall drop in overdose deaths statewide.**[19]
  - The program screens all Rhode Island inmates for opioid use disorders and provides medication-assisted treatment for those who need it. Upon release, they are connected with treatment resources in the community.
  - The study showed a 61 percent decrease in post-incarceration overdose deaths, which contributed to a 12 percent reduction in overdose deaths in the state's overall population.
  - The study, led by Rhode Island health commissioner Nicole Alexander-Scott, showed that providing treatment to everyone who is incarcerated is a promising strategy to address the opioid epidemic, an approach that other states are working to emulate.
- **In Delaware, state officials reached out to Saloner and the Johns Hopkins Bloomberg School of Public Health and the Bloomberg American Health Initiative for help after overdose fatalities in the state jumped by 12 percent in 2017.**[20] Saloner's July 2018 report, called "A Blueprint for Transforming Opioid Use Disorder Treatment in Delaware," outlined these steps:
  - *Increase the capacity of the treatment system.* This includes, among other things, providing rapid intake and assessment, treatment with medication and counseling, peer mentorship services, and access to chronic disease management. This strategy recognizes that the "gateway to care" has multiple entry points, ranging from hospitals and urgent care centers to police officers, recovery programs, family, and physicians.
  - *Engage high-risk populations in treatment.* This strategy includes offering treatment through the Department of Corrections, upgrading three existing opioid withdrawal management centers, and setting standards for hospital-based treatment and peer support.
  - *Creating incentives for quality care,* ensuring that there is adequate and consistent reimbursement for high-quality services to treat opioid use disorder.
  - *Using data to guide reform and monitor progress.* This strategy brings together multi-agency data in order to understand system effectiveness, opportunities for improvement, and treatment capacity.

- **In West Virginia, the state has worked to develop a Medicaid 1115 waiver that will build on legislative and other governmental efforts to combat substance use.**
  - The Medicaid 1115 waiver permits the state to increase the availability of substance use prevention and treatment services—essentially creating a continuum of care that incorporates screening, brief intervention, and referral to treatment; coverage for methadone treatment; comprehensive initiatives for naloxone to reduce overdose deaths; peer support; and short-term residential treatment. (West Virginia's Medicaid 1115 waiver program is described in detail in Chapter 11, "Driving Innovation Through Medicaid.")
- **In the community of Huntington, W.Va., health officials have joined together to embrace "Huntington's Road to Recovery" initiatives that provide community-wide and cross-sector solutions to the opioid crisis and emphasize the power of partnerships.**
  - Since 2009, Huntington's Road to Recovery efforts have engaged medical, educational, and social service providers, support groups, child advocates, first responders, and addiction/treatment specialists. For instance, Marshall University formed a Substance Use Recovery Coalition in 2015 to guide its efforts to fight the opioid crisis; in 2017, health officials developed a quick response team to contact individuals who had overdosed in the previous three days to discuss treatment options; in 2018, Hoops Family Children's Hospital developed a program to provide addiction treatment services to postpartum women while their babies recover from neonatal abstinence syndrome.
- **In Kentucky, officials have determined that confronting the opioid epidemic requires both supply- and demand-side policy solutions and interventions.**
  - Supply-side interventions included the mandatory use of prescription drug monitoring programs, which the CDC has called "among the most promising state-level interventions to monitor and improve opioid prescribing, inform clinical practices, and protect patients at risk."[21] The Kentucky program has been modified several times to increase its effectiveness and appears to be working well; one recent change restricts prescriptions for controlled substances to a three-day supply.
  - On the demand side, interventions include prevention education for patients and prescribers. One example involves educating physicians on how to reduce the length of pain medication prescriptions after emergency room visits and surgery, and in some cases to replace addictive drugs with nonsteroidal anti-inflammatories. Another statewide change

included reducing cash-only buprenorphine clinics that weren't providing high-quality treatment, such as behavioral counseling.

- In addition, Kentucky has a Medicaid 1115 waiver that includes coverage for residential treatment services, which were not previously available to people suffering from opioid addiction.

Despite these promising programs and strategies, Waller warned that controlling the opioid epidemic requires controlling something bigger: the multilayered, complicated issue of addiction. And treating addiction, he acknowledged, is filled with uncertainties.

"Some things we're going to try, and they will fail," he said. "And when they fail, we pull them back, and then we try something else. And then we evaluate the data and the science on the outside of it, so that we start to implement programs that have sustainability. That are humane. That have the capability to actually stabilize not the disease of an opioid use disorder—but of addiction."

A Final Word

At the opening plenary of the 2018 *Sharing Knowledge* conference, Robert K. Ross, MD, president and chief executive officer of the California Endowment, noted that when RWJF "declared that a Culture of Health was the way to go— that was the declaration of a moon shot." And although he admitted that he doesn't know "exactly the 10 steps to get to a Culture of Health, all of us knows what happens when you don't have it. You get an opioid epidemic, school shootings, you get Ferguson, Missouri."

Indeed, the opioid epidemic demonstrates just how far many regions are from achieving a Culture of Health. Advancing health equity requires addressing the multifaceted drivers of the opioid epidemic through innovative multisector programs that shift the emphasis from punishment and stigma to upstream solutions. Driven by an understanding of the unique cultural and historical contexts of their communities, front-line advocates and policymakers at all levels will need to collaborate on a package of well-coordinated strategies.

There is a glimmer of hope that ongoing efforts are beginning to show results. In July 2019, the CDC reported that drug overdose deaths had declined by around 5 percent in the previous year, the first such drop since 1990. However, another sobering statistic revealed the continuing complexity of the problem. According to the CDC, the decline in drug overdose deaths was due almost completely to fewer deaths from prescription opioid painkillers, while fatal overdoses involving other drugs, such as fentanyl, continued to rise.[22]

This is a crucial moment to identify, learn from, and promote community-based approaches that address multiple systems and sectors. For example, RWJF has recently funded the Pew Charitable Trusts to develop a Call for Proposals that will fund evaluations of existing equity-focused, community innovations that address the opioid epidemic.[23] Through evaluation and widespread dissemination of promising or successful community-led approaches, the underlying causes and community conditions that negatively impact well-being and health equity can be recognized and transformed.

Chapter 7 Spotlight: Rural Addiction: A Perfect Storm, a Nod to Grandma, Pills for Cash

A core question about the unfolding of the opioid epidemic begs for an answer: How and why is it such a devastating problem in rural areas?

Granted, the documented pattern of overprescribing in rural states is part of the answer, as is a lack of access to health care insurance and the long distances between homes and medical care facilities and physicians. But experts know it is more complicated than these combined explanations. Asked during an interview to provide his personal observations on this question, James Becker's unvarnished answer goes straight to his lived experiences in West Virginia, reflecting decades of treating addiction in rural communities that are caught in what he called "the perfect storm":

"Appalachia was in a perfect storm for this. Culturally, people in Appalachia were very comfortable with taking pills. The way health care has been set up here over the years, you had a lot of small, one-doctor and two-doctor medical practices. People went to those doctors for just about everything, and it usually involved either getting a prescription for an antibiotic or a pain pill or a shot. And there were doctors who were very liberal about giving people a shot of penicillin, a prescription for Zithromax, some quick fix. Whether it was truly indicated or not, people expected it.

"So there's this heavy reliance on taking a pill—and that led people to feel very comfortable with the fact that you can take a pill. And not only that, but Grandma would give you a pill if she thought you needed something. So this idea of self-medicating or sharing medication is kind of a culturally accepted behavior."

In hard times, rural people with access to prescriptions sometimes turn their pills into cash. Becker continued:

"So you have this cultural background, and then you have the economic downturn, and you have the isolation in communities and the counties that we're in—whether we're talking about eastern Kentucky, southern Pennsylvania, southern Ohio, all of West Virginia, eastern Tennessee. These counties were heavily relying on extractive industries, and when that crumbled and their employment couldn't be had, people didn't want to leave. They were strongly attached to their community and to their family, but they didn't have a way to make a living.

"If you had an injury that would justify a doctor giving you a prescription for a medicine that would be paid for by insurance of some sort, then you had a way of getting a bottle of pills that had street value. You could let people know you had a bottle of Percocet [the brand name of oxycodone] and each pill might be worth $5 or $10 a tablet. People would call and say, 'Can I get 10 Percocets from you?' and they would come over and give you $100 for it.

"Well, that $100 might pay your car payment. So it turned this struggling economy into an economy with a large, illegitimate economy running within it. It was all cash and money moving around to buy pills. And when the controls on prescriptions started, that took away the prescriptions and then the supply to the point that people were more willing to use heroin—which is dirt cheap. Around here, a dose of heroin to get you through the day is going to cost you the same thing as a pack of cigarettes: five bucks."

Achieving Health Equity for Immigrants and Their Children

Duncan Lawrence, PhD, Executive Director, Immigration Policy Lab, Stanford University

Karthick Ramakrishnan, PhD, Founding Director, Center for Social Innovation; Professor of Public Policy and Political Science, University of California, Riverside

Katherine Yun, MD, MHS, Assistant Professor of Pediatrics, University of Pennsylvania Perelman School of Medicine; Faculty, Policy Lab, Children's Hospital of Philadelphia

Immigrants and their children represent a quarter (27%) of the U.S. population, approximately 86.4 million people.[1] This heterogeneous group of people—who may be documented or undocumented—includes migrants seeking to join family, accept jobs, or pursue opportunity and refugees fleeing violence, war, and persecution, many of whom may be seeking asylum in the United States. Many of their children know no other home but the United States.

Immigration has been a hot-button issue for the public and policymakers of all political persuasions for some time. What can be considered "immigration policy" includes a range of rules and procedures that determine whether immigrants are allowed to enter the United States and how they are treated once here, as well as other government policy, guidelines, and practices that touch their lives. All of these may affect immigrant health, noted Duncan Lawrence of Stanford University. "There is clear evidence that immigration policy, whether in health care or policies that protect parents and individuals from deportation, impacts the health and well-being of children in immigrant families and immigrant families in general."

Recently, these issues have drawn heightened attention as the current administration has put policies in place that separate families at the southern border,

Culture of Health in Practice, Alonzo L. Plough. Oxford University Press (2020) © Robert Wood Johnson Foundation
DOI: 10.1093/oso/9780190071400.001.0001

require long periods of detention, and step up deportation and other enforcement measures.

The contributors to this chapter describe today's immigrants, how immigration is framed in public discourse and policymaking, and how public policies support or undermine the health and well-being of immigrants and their children. Karthick Ramakrishnan cuts through familiar rhetoric to inform our understanding of the immigrant population and how it is affected by both federal and state policy. Katherine Yun addresses health care access for immigrant children while Lawrence describes policy changes that have a positive impact on the health of children in immigrant families.

A Brief List of Immigration-Related Terms*

- **Undocumented immigrants**: Foreign-born individuals without a legal right to be in or to remain in the United States. Undocumented immigrants (also referred to as unauthorized immigrants) may have entered:
  - Illegally, without border inspection
  - Legally, and then "overstayed" a visa or temporary legal status after the expiration date
- **Refugees**: Individuals living outside the United States who meet international and U.S. refugee criteria (demonstration of persecution or fear of persecution due to race, religion, nationality, political opinion, or membership in a particular social group)
- **Asylee**: Refugees already in the United States or at a port of entry who are seeking or have been granted asylum in the United States. Asylees may apply for permanent resident status after living in the United States for a year after receiving asylum status.
- **Lawfully present**: People allowed to stay legally in the United States, which includes refugees and asylees, as well as:
  - **Temporary residents**: Tourists, business people, foreign government officials and journalists, students, temporary workers, etc.
  - **Permanent residents**: People holding a "green card" that allows them to live and work in the United States indefinitely
- **Visas**: There are approximately 185 different visa types, in two main categories:
  - **Non-immigrant visas** for temporary visits (e.g., H-1B for those in specialty occupations working here temporarily and H-4 for their spouses and children)

- *Immigrant visas*, including family-based (relatives of U.S. citizens and lawful permanent residents), employment-based (individuals with extraordinary ability in various areas, researchers, executives, those with special skills, and others), adoption, diversity (from countries with low immigration rates), special immigrants (e.g., Iraqi or Afghan translators/interpreters), and others
- *Naturalized citizens*: Foreign-born people who become U.S. citizens with all of the rights of citizenship except eligibility to be president or vice president. Generally a person may apply for citizenship after five years as a permanent resident.

*U.S. government terms and definitions are used here. Other groups may use different definitions.

Portrait of American Immigrants

What is the reality of the immigrant population in America? How many immigrants are living in the United States, where do they come from, and how do they arrive? What is their legal status? And what is their health status upon arrival and after living in this country? The answers to these questions offer a fuller picture of a population whose residency status engenders much controversy and misunderstanding.

Record Numbers of Immigrants

In 2016 the number of immigrants living in the United States reached a record 43.7 million, representing 13.5 percent of the U.S. population. That percentage is second only to the peak of the immigration wave in the late 19th and early 20th centuries, when immigrants represented 14.8 percent of the population (9.2 million). The percentage subsequently dropped under a national quota system that sought to limit or block immigration from regions other than Western and Northern Europe, especially Asia, until it was replaced by the 1965 Immigration and Nationality Act. At the lowest point in 1970, immigrants represented just 4.7 percent of the U.S. population. After that, the percentage began to increase steadily.[2]

Millions of children, whether born in the United States or not, are part of immigrant families. According to the Urban Institute, as of 2017, 18.6 million children (25.9% of all U.S. children) had at least one immigrant parent, with 7.2 million having only noncitizen parents. Close to half (49.2%) of all children living in California had at least one immigrant parent. Most children in immigrant families (16.3 million) were themselves born in the United States and are citizens.[3]

Countries and Regions of Origin

In 2016, South and East Asian immigrants constituted 27 percent of immigrants *living* in the United States, and Mexican immigrants accounted for 26 percent. Other regions followed: Central and South America (15%), Europe and Canada (13%), the Caribbean (10%), and the Middle East and sub-Saharan Africa (4% each).

India was the top country of origin for immigrants *arriving* in 2016, with China and Mexico close behind. The number of Asian immigrants has outpaced those from Latin America every year since 2010, and today more immigrants come from China than from Mexico. In fact, immigration from Mexico is a net negative now, with more people returning than arriving.[4]

"This shows how out-of-touch our rhetoric on immigration is with the reality of how things are actually playing out on the ground," said Karthick Ramakrishnan of the University of California, Riverside, whose research focus includes U.S. immigration policy and politics. Mexico, however, remains the conduit for increasing numbers of undocumented immigrants from El Salvador, Guatemala, and Honduras.[5]

The majority of Asian immigrants arrive on a family-based visa, not on an employment visa as many believe, according to Ramakrishnan. Overall, individuals with family-based visas account for the largest proportion of immigrants, compared with those holding employment- and diversity-based visas and with refugees and asylum-seekers.[6]

Legal Status

Just under a quarter (24%) of immigrants in the United States are undocumented—10.7 million people, representing 3.3 percent of the U.S. population. Some 45 percent are naturalized U.S. citizens, while 27 percent are lawful permanent residents ("green card" holders) and 5 percent are lawful temporary residents. The number of undocumented immigrants has decreased from a record high in 2007, primarily as a result of the decline in immigrants from Mexico.[7]

The Asian undocumented population, however, more than tripled between 2001 and 2015; as of 2018, about one in seven Asian immigrants is undocumented, according to Ramakrishnan. During the same period, those from Central America tripled and those from Africa more than doubled.[8] Presumably, most undocumented Asian and African immigrants have overstayed their visas, but few data exist on the type of visa with which they arrived or their demographics (age, occupation, etc.).

Many undocumented immigrants have lived in the United States for long periods of time—an average of 14.8 years, as of 2016. Nearly half live in three states: California (24%), Texas (11%), and New York (10%). Grouped by region, about two-thirds live in the West (34%) and the South (33%), 21 percent in the Northeast, and 11 percent in the Midwest.[9]

Health Status

Generalizations about the health status of immigrants are often inaccurate because the population is so diverse. [10] For example, certain birth outcomes are better among children of Mexican immigrants and worse among Indian immigrants, compared to the overall U.S. population.

Nonetheless, research tends to show that the health status of immigrants arriving in the United States is better than that of both native-born Americans overall and native-born members of the same ethnic or racial group—a pattern often called the "immigrant paradox." Immigrants have a lower incidence of all cancers, fewer chronic conditions, lower obesity rates, and lower infant mortality rates, and are less likely to die from cardiovascular disease and all cancers combined. Immigrants are also less likely than people born in the United States to be depressed or to misuse alcohol. (The immigrant paradox is exemplified by the Hispanic mortality paradox, the finding that Hispanics in the United States live longer, on average, than the overall population, despite their greater health risks, possibly because of certain features in their culture. (That topic is explored in detail in Chapter 1, "Incorporating 'Culture' Within a Culture of Health.")

The explanations that have been suggested for the immigrant paradox include "selection effect" (healthier individuals may be more likely to migrate than those who are less healthy), "salmon bias" (sicker immigrants are more likely to return to their home countries), and social and cultural factors that support healthy diets and lifestyles. This last factor also may explain why immigrant health status tends to decline over time in the United States as immigrants and their children adopt American practices such as diets heavy in convenience food, increased alcohol and drug use, and less involvement with family. A further explanation for these health declines over time may be that poor and low-skilled immigrants often work in jobs with physical dangers and risky chemical exposure (e.g., in nail salons).

The generally younger age of the immigrant population—many are working-age taxpayers—is a plus for the Medicare Trust Fund. Immigrant contributions to the Trust Fund, compared to the cost of care paid by Medicare for immigrants, netted a total surplus of $115.2 billion from 2002 through 2009. Immigrants accounted for 14.7 percent of total Medicare contributions in 2009, yet just 7.9 percent of expenditures.[11]

The Policy Landscape

Government policy touching on immigration includes a wide range of laws, rules, regulations, and practices at the federal, state, and local levels. The framing, stipulations, and enforcement of government policy influence the lives and health of immigrants both directly and indirectly.

Why Policy Framing Matters

How immigration policy is framed can be quite powerful, noted Ramakrishnan, who believes that "framing matters as much as or sometimes even more than the demographic facts." He highlighted these frames:

- Using the word "amnesty" will reduce support for pro-integration policies (measures that promote and reinforce the inclusion of immigrants into the economic, social, and cultural fabric of the country).
- Framing a policy as focused on children will increase support for pro-integration policies.
- There is more support for integration rather than deportation when talking about immigrants who have lived in this country for long periods of time, say 10 or 20 years.
- "Chain migration" is a pejorative term for "family reunification," the official policy that allows green card holders or legal U.S. residents to sponsor a family member for immigration.
- Chain migration is linked to another negative concept, the "population bomb," which is supposedly ignited by one immigrant, then two, and increasing exponentially. "It's a very misleading and anxiety-inducing metaphor for legal immigration," said Ramakrishnan.
- Another term that labels immigrants as problems is "public charge"—the idea that, by using government benefits such as Medicaid or Section 8 housing, an immigrant is a drain on the United States. The health implications of being labeled a public charge, or even threatened with that label, are explored below.

"This is part of a larger effort to portray immigrants, including legal immigrants for the first time, as harmful to the United States," said Ramakrishnan. He noted that the messaging from the White House echoes that of organizations advocating restrictions on immigration.

Federal Policies

The federal government, particularly the White House, has significant power over immigration policy; the president can issue executive orders to impel enforcement in a variety of ways. The Obama administration was viewed as enforcement-heavy at its start, said Ramakrishnan, but later moved toward an approach that favored integration.

The Trump administration has expanded enforcement inside U.S. borders, conducting administrative arrests (arrests for civil violations of immigration law) at routine Department of Homeland Security check-ins, which can prompt further investigation or deportation. A number of other actions have been under consideration by the Trump administration, including revoking the ability of some holders of H-4 visas (spouses of H-1B workers in the United States who are awaiting green card approval) from working and rescinding the ability to renew an H-1B visa more than twice. Ramakrishnan also noted that there has been a "dramatic slow-down" in the naturalization process leading to citizenship and in the processing of applications for green cards.

State Policies

For many years, states have acted as laboratories for innovative ideas and practices that eventually emerge at the federal level. Women's suffrage, smoking bans, minimum wage laws, and other movements began locally, grew at a state level, and then pushed to the federal level, Ramakrishnan observed. The states can exert similar influence over immigration issues, although they vary greatly in their approach.

Ramakrishnan described how various types of "state citizenship" can affect an immigrant's access to rights and benefits:

- *Regressive* state citizenship—states take away rights guaranteed at the federal level, as in the Jim Crow South. Some of these policies are likely to be challenged in federal court.
- *Reinforcing* state citizenship—states use federal entitlement categories in ways that control access to rights and benefits at the state level. An example is Arizona, the first state to enact broad and strict anti-illegal immigration legislation (2010), garnering national and international attention and controversy, as well as strong legal challenges.

- *Progressive* state citizenship—states expand rights beyond those provided at the federal level, as in California, which has measures in place to promote the integration of immigrants.

"Though we think of immigration policy as something that the federal government has purview over, states have become centers of making immigration policy," said Stanford's Lawrence, "as they increasingly adopt policies that affect immigrants, asylum seekers, and refugees."

> It's important not to view immigration only through a nationwide lens but to understand that what's going on in states and communities makes a difference. —Duncan Lawrence

While immigrant access to services is increasingly restricted at the federal level, some states are taking the opposite approach and making benefits and services more accessible. Although research evidence is mixed, newly arrived immigrants do not, in general, seek to situate themselves in states with the most robust set of benefits; rather, they mainly use personal networks, often linked to jobs, to determine where they will live.

Key Influences on Immigrant Health

Immigrants in America vary greatly by country of origin (with associated cultural practices and history), arrival story, immigration status, work-related skill set, family connections, state of residence, and so on. All of these factors will affect the health of immigrants and their children, as well as their ability to obtain appropriate health care as needed.

Despite individual differences, several overarching themes are key to considering how policy can impact immigrant health:

- *Policies that extend public health insurance coverage* to more categories of immigrants are a step toward greater health equity.
- *Policies and programs that go beyond insurance coverage* to further meaningful access to health care help ensure that immigrants actually secure the health services they need and to which they are entitled.
- *The mixed immigration status among members of many immigrant families* can foster anxiety, confusion, and an unwillingness to access benefits for eligible family members. "It's a very different health system experience for U.S. citizen children of lawful permanent residents than for those with at least one undocumented parent," Lawrence observed.

- *Policies that facilitate the integration of immigrants* have spillover effects on immigrant health. For example, granting driver's licenses to undocumented immigrants will increase their ability to keep health service appointments for themselves and their children.
- *The debate playing out between states and between states and the federal government* as to whether government policy should promote the integration of immigrants or impede it by restricting access to benefits and services will have direct and indirect effects on the health of immigrants and their children. For example, children's health will be affected when a parent finds it difficult to obtain employment. Fear of parental deportation may lead to chronic school absenteeism and other long-term impacts on child development.

Access to Health Care for Immigrant Children

A recurring theme in health circles is that access to comprehensive, quality health care often presents challenges for children in immigrant families. "No matter where you work in health equity and health disparities, you are going to intersect with immigrant families," said Katherine Yun of Children's Hospital of Philadelphia. Yun's research and clinical work focus on the well-being of children in those families.

Although many factors may be barriers to care, community leaders cite "access to health insurance and to language services as the two most important when it comes to getting health care for children," said Yun.

Health Insurance Coverage

Lack of insurance not only imposes a health care burden on children but also a social and emotional burden. Children whose health needs are not met may miss school, not participate in sports, and generally lack connections with ordinary childhood and adolescent activities.

Medicaid and the Children's Health Insurance Program (CHIP), which covers children in families who earn somewhat more than the maximum allowed under Medicaid, provide a solid base of health coverage in all states for low-income children and pregnant women who are U.S. citizens. All but two states cover children from families with incomes up to at least 200 percent of the federal poverty level ($41,500 for a family of three in 2018). Some 19 states cover children with family income at or above 300 percent.[12] In 2018, 34 states covered pregnant women up to at least 300 percent of the federal poverty level.

In the 36 states and the District of Columbia that have implemented Medicaid expansion under the Affordable Care Act as of April 2019,[13] eligibility for parents and other adults has significantly increased; in those without Medicaid expansion, eligibility is very limited. As an indicator of the health-promoting nature of Medicaid, mean infant mortality in Medicaid-expansion states declined significantly more than in states that did not expand Medicaid.[14]

The situation is more complicated for immigrant children and families. At the federal level:

- Children born in the United States to immigrant parents are themselves citizens and eligible for Medicaid/CHIP if otherwise eligible under the rules of the state in which they reside.
- Lawful permanent residents who have resided in the United States for more than five years, refugees, and asylees are eligible for Medicaid/CHIP if otherwise eligible under the rules of the state in which they reside.
- As a result of the 2009 CHIP reauthorization, states have the option of expanding coverage to all lawfully residing children and pregnant women, which includes lawful permanent residents and lawfully present temporary residents, regardless of how long they have lived in the United States. As of January 2018, 33 states have expanded coverage to lawfully residing children and to lawfully residing pregnant women.[15]
- There is generally no routine Medicaid coverage for undocumented children or adults, except in limited emergency situations.
- Eligibility for select childhood nutrition programs—such as the Special Supplemental Nutrition Program for Women, Infants, and Children (WIC) and school breakfasts and lunches—is determined without regard to immigration status.

Other policies important for immigrant families are state- and municipality-based programs that expand insurance eligibility even further.

- Some states, including New York and Washington, use state funds to expand coverage to a wider group of resident immigrants. New York's Child Health Plus program is available to all children in the state regardless of immigration status or income. Low-income pregnant women can receive Medicaid irrespective of immigration status.
- California currently covers undocumented immigrant children under Medi-Cal, the state Medicaid program, until they are 19 years old. In his first state budget proposal (January 2019) the new governor of California, Gavin Newsom, included expanding that coverage until the age of 26, under terms similar to those in the Affordable Care Act.[16]

- Also in January 2019, New York City mayor Bill de Blasio announced that the city will spend up to $100 million annually to expand health care access to low-income city residents, including undocumented immigrants, who do not have insurance.[17] The program expects to serve approximately 600,000 residents, half of whom lack insurance due to their immigration status. It includes access to primary care physicians, mental health services, and prescription drug coverage.

Will Public Charge Rule Changes Reduce the Use of Benefits by Immigrants?

Even when they are eligible, many immigrants choose not to apply for, or to use, public health insurance, due to concerns about being labeled a "public charge."[18] The fear is that it could impact their eligibility (or that of a family member) for a green card or other immigration applications, or increase their risk of deportation.

Until August 2019, the emphasis in the public charge assessment was on the likelihood that an applicant for public benefits would become *primarily dependent* on the government for support through use of cash assistance, such as Temporary Assistance for Needy Families (TANF, a program for very low-income families with children), Supplemental Security Income (SSI, for aged, blind, or disabled people with little or no income), or long-term institutional care. The use of government-funded health care, nutrition, or housing programs had traditionally been viewed as instrumental to community health, safety, and productivity, and not typically counted against an applicant.

On October 10, 2018, the Department of Homeland Security (DHS) proposed a new public charge rule. In contrast to the previous rule, the proposed regulation defined a person as a public charge who only *uses* a government program. Medicaid, Supplemental Nutrition Assistance Program (SNAP, formerly known as food stamps), Section 8 housing, the low-income subsidy for the Medicare Part D prescription drug benefit, as well as all forms of cash aid, including state and local assistance programs, would be included in the assessment. A total of 266,077 comments[19] were submitted during the public comment period ending December 10, 2018.

On August 14, 2019, DHS published the new rule, *Inadmissibility on Public Charge Grounds*, in the Federal Register, including a reference to the strong opposition expressed by most people who had commented on the proposed rule: "[w]hile some commenters provided support for the rule, the vast majority of commenters opposed the rule."[20]

The new regulation targets legal immigrants applying for a green card by employing a considerably more burdensome standard than the previous rule in determining whether a green card applicant has the financial means for personal support. Under the rule, immigrants will be denied a green card if they are considered *likely* to use any of the government programs noted above as specifically designated in the proposed rule (Medicaid, SNAP, housing vouchers, Medicare Part D subsidy, cash assistance programs, etc.). A number of federal programs are *not* included in the public charge inadmissibility determination, including WIC, CHIP, school breakfast/lunch programs, and Head Start. The rule will not apply to use of Medicaid by pregnant women and children, emergency Medicaid, Medicaid received for services provided under the Individuals with Disabilities Education Act (IDEA), or to benefits received by certain members of the U.S. Armed Forces and their families, refugees and asylees, and specified others. The effective date for the new rule is October 15, 2019, although legal challenges are expected. It is not clear if these legal challenges will restrict implementation.

The change in regulation is likely to influence the willingness of immigrants, even those not affected by the rule, to enroll in programs for which they or their children are eligible—what is referred to as the "chilling effect." As an example, when word of the proposed change was leaked (though nothing official had yet been issued), immigrant mothers began to dis-enroll from WIC and other such programs, worried that participation would have an adverse effect on themselves or someone else in their families.

With announcement of the implementation of the new rule, advocacy organizations believe that as many as 26 million immigrants living legally in the United States will reassess whether to continue use of government benefits due to their fear of the effect of that use on their immigration status.[21]

Language Access

The inability to communicate with one's health care provider can have serious negative consequences in terms of access to care, quality of care, health status, safety, medication overdoses, and so on.[22] This issue cuts across all immigrant groups.

> *You could be a highly trained engineer from China or you could be an immigrant from China with less than a high school education. If you don't speak English proficiently, your children could have very similar experiences when it comes to seeking health care. —Katherine Yun*

About 9 percent of the U.S. population age 5 or older (25.9 million people) is considered "limited English proficient" (i.e., speaking English less than "very well"), according to the U.S. Census Bureau. About 20 percent of the population speaks a foreign language at home.[23]

The 1964 Civil Rights Act provides the legal framework for ensuring that health care providers who receive federal funding via Medicaid, Medicare, and other public programs offer equitable services regardless of any language barrier and provide interpreter services for patients who do not speak English. As a result, health systems are increasingly likely to offer qualified interpreter services either in-person or by video or telephone. However, children and families with limited English proficiency continue to experience language barriers when seeking health care.

Even when such services are available, health professionals may not be trained in working with a professional interpreter and may instead communicate through family members. Nonclinical staff also must have access to interpreters and receive training to work with them effectively. A 2017 "mystery shopper" study in which a bilingual "parent" called developmental pediatrics programs affiliated with U.S. children's hospitals requesting an appointment for his child found that less information was provided to the caller when the caller spoke Spanish than when he spoke English and that 31 percent did not provide language accommodations.[24]

In addition, while clinicians may consider themselves "proficient" or "fluent" in another language and able to conduct clinic visits with non-English-speaking patients, research has found that self-reported language ability does not reliably predict actual, tested ability in the clinical setting.[25] Some form of credentialing would ensure that providers are, in fact, able to provide care in another language.

Language barriers may be particularly distressing for children in need of mental or behavioral health care.[26] Access to appropriate mental health care is an issue for all children in the United States due to barriers that include stigma, shortages of child and adolescent psychologists and psychiatrists, and racial and ethnic disparities in the availability of treatment options.[27] For children from immigrant families, the obstacles presented by language disparities can make accessing appropriate services especially daunting. "Not all refugee and immigrant children experience significant emotional distress or have a mental illness such that they would seek or need formal mental health care," Yun said, "but some do, and for those children access can be very challenging."

Policies Proven to Improve Health

Immigrant children, of course, have the same health care needs as other children, but they are also subject to physical and mental health challenges related to their own immigration status and that of their parents. When governments and communities adopt policies to protect, support, and welcome immigrants, there is striking evidence that their children are more likely to thrive. Lawrence and researchers at the Immigration Policy Lab evaluated two policy changes, one federal and one state, that demonstrate a positive impact on the health of children from immigrant families.

Parental DACA Eligibility: Reducing Anxiety in Children

The status and future of the 11 million undocumented immigrants are the subject of fierce debate. The introduction of Deferred Action for Childhood Arrivals (DACA) in 2012 offered an opportunity for a quasi-experimental study investigating the impact of parents' tenuous immigration status on the health of their citizen children.

About DACA

On June 15, 2012, President Barack Obama launched DACA, a program that allows young people who came to the United States as children to be "lawfully present" without threat of deportation and to be able to apply for driver's licenses and work permits. It does not confer official legal status nor does it provide a pathway to citizenship. To apply for DACA an applicant had to be at least 15 and less than 31 years of age on June 15, 2012, and to have lived continuously in the United States since June 15, 2007. Close to 800,000 individuals initially received DACA status. More than 200,000 U.S. citizen children had a parent eligible for DACA at program launch. [28]

By September 2017, about 70,000 DACA participants had not renewed their benefits or had had renewal applications denied, and another 40,000 had obtained green cards.[29] Thus, about 690,000 young adults had DACA status (nearly 80 percent of whom were of Mexican origin) when the Trump administration announced plans to end the program and subsequently refused to support several bills in Congress designed to address DACA's future. In January 2018, a federal judge in California issued an injunction that allowed individuals with DACA to renew their status, and judges in New York and Washington followed suit. No new applications are being taken.

How DACA Changed Children's Lives

DACA's specific start date offered a convenient way to establish comparison groups; an individual who was even one day older than 31 on June 15, 2012, was ineligible. Using Oregon Medicaid data, researchers were able to identify quasi-treatment and quasi-control groups of women whose birth date (just after or just before this cut point) made them eligible for DACA or not, despite being almost the same age.

The researchers compared Medicaid claims for adjustment and anxiety disorders among children before and after DACA was launched. They found:

- No difference in diagnoses among children whose mothers became eligible for DACA, compared to those who did not, before DACA was announced.
- A drop of more than 50 percent in adjustment and anxiety disorders in children of DACA-eligible mothers after DACA was announced.

Although the positive impact of DACA eligibility on children's mental health was not surprising, "the magnitude of the effect is really substantial," said Lawrence, who stressed that "policymakers need to realize that they can have a massive impact on the health and well-being of kids simply by affecting the status of those children's parents. It's a really powerful policy lever." A pediatrician who works with the team added, "There's no medication or therapy that I could provide to kids systematically that would have this type of impact."

The study's authors summarized the findings in this way: "Parents' unauthorized status is thus a substantial barrier to normal child development and perpetuates health inequalities through the intergenerational transmission of disadvantage."[30]

In work underway in early 2019, sociologists with the Stanford team are interviewing DACA recipients and undocumented parents to understand how undocumented status affects health care access and parents' ability to feel they are providing a safe and secure environment for their children. The team also is conducting DACA impact studies in California and New York and hopes to use this model to examine policies in all 50 states.

Study findings have been included in congressional testimony and supported California's lawsuit seeking an injunction against revoking DACA. Thus, said Lawrence, the study "has been used by those who are trying to make a case, either legally or from an advocacy framework, about why DACA should be extended and not cancelled by the current administration."

The Oregon Experiment: Expanding Prenatal Care

Emergency Medicaid covers labor and delivery care for undocumented immigrants and those lawfully present in the United States for less than five years. Unlike standard Medicaid, it does not provide comprehensive coverage. Prenatal care is not included, and coverage for the mother generally ends at childbirth. The children, however, are eligible for standard Medicaid/CHIP as U.S.-born citizens. At least 16 states extend prenatal care to the population eligible for Emergency Medicaid under CHIP's "unborn child option," which allows states to cover the unborn child (who will be a U.S. citizen) from conception to birth.

Extending Prenatal Coverage Improves Health

Between April 2008 and October 2013, Oregon extended prenatal care to undocumented immigrant women (called Emergency Medicaid Plus), introducing the coverage in a staggered rollout by county. The Stanford and Oregon Health & Science University (OHSU) researchers who evaluated the impact of this inclusive health care policy found that immigrant women's use of prenatal care increased dramatically.[31,32]

- The detection of pregnancy complications and high-risk conditions (e.g., pre-existing Type 2 diabetes, hypertensive disorders of pregnancy, and history of preterm birth) improved significantly.
- On average, pregnant women had 7.2 more prenatal visits, and diabetes screenings increased by 61 percent.
- Prenatal ultrasounds increased by 74 percent.

The impact on children was also substantial:

- Infants were healthier; infant mortality and the incidence of extremely low birthweight babies decreased significantly.
- Vaccination rates increased, not only providing immunization protection, but also indicating that mothers were engaging with the health care system and using preventive care—developments with positive implications for children's future health.

As of early 2019, Stanford and OHSU researchers were analyzing the cost of extending Medicaid coverage to determine the cost-effectiveness of this policy change.

Where to Look Next

Clearly, both federal and state policy have important impacts on the health of immigrants and their children. Although federal policy may have turned in a more restrictive direction in recent years, a number of states have taken an opposing path, perhaps boding well for the future of immigrant health.

Several areas of inquiry suggest other ways to understand this complex subject. It is important to note, however, that trying to identify the effects of policy on the undocumented population is challenging, because it is often difficult for researchers to determine who is undocumented. There are also ethical concerns about states sharing data on their undocumented populations and researchers using those data without increasing the risk of deportation for study populations.

- *There has been relatively little research on the large population of asylum seekers uncertain about their future,* according to Lawrence, who hypothesizes that the situation most likely "has long-term negative consequences for mental well-being, economic stability, and so on. The asylum process and growing backlog of cases deserve more attention as a public health issue."
- *Longitudinal work would further understanding of the impact of current policies on child development in immigrant families,* such as the effect on educational performance. Tracking immigrant cohorts over time is a "missing piece of the puzzle," said Lawrence.
- *More knowledge about the impact of various inclusive and exclusive state-level insurance coverage policies on child development and long-term health outcomes* would contribute to understanding their value.
- *Another avenue worth exploring is the potential health challenges that children in immigrant families might face as a result of their long-term exposure to stress.*
- *There is a need to study how to implement solutions.* "There's been amazing pioneering work showing where we have deficiencies and disparities," said Yun. "We need to figure out, in a meaningful and systematic way, how to address those and how to scale up any solutions that are promising so that they exist for immigrants in the real world and not just on the pages of a journal."

A Final Word

Many immigrants and their children in the United States face a daunting array of stressors, demands, legal issues, health risks, economic barriers, and other obstacles to good health. Ensuring that these families are supported requires health care providers, policymakers, and community leaders to acknowledge the myriad factors influencing the health of their immigrant constituents. It is a path that will improve well-being for immigrants, while offering benefits more broadly as we work toward health equity.

9

Climate Change, Environmental Stressors, and Resilience

Liesel Ashley Ritchie, PhD., Associate Director, Center for the Study of Disasters and Extreme Events, and Associate Professor, Department of Sociology, Oklahoma State University

Elizabeth C. Yeampierre, Executive Director, UPROSE

The aftermath of weather-related disasters in Houston, Puerto Rico, the Virgin Islands, and California. . . . The consequences of human-driven environmental catastrophes such as the poisoned water crisis in Flint, Mich., and the Deepwater Horizon oil spill . . . the health impacts of diminished air quality leading to asthma and rising temperatures leading to heat-related illnesses and deaths . . .

These are just a few of the environmental stressors that confront a world impacted by climate change and disasters. Today, more than ever, ensuring that communities are resilient enough to withstand the aftermath, consequences, and health impacts of these kinds of crises is foundational for building a Culture of Health.[1]

As seen repeatedly over the last few decades, adverse environmental conditions expose millions of people to deadly heat waves, severe drought, nuclear waste, oil spills, coal ash, and other extreme environmental challenges. The consequences are dire, and exacerbate existing health inequalities.

These adverse conditions will only grow more urgent in the future, doing their greatest damage to the world's poorest and most vulnerable populations. That puts people with chronic health conditions, the economically marginalized, communities of color, and those who live in disadvantaged communities most in harm's way.[2]

"We know that these disasters hit communities that are suffering from chronic stressors much harder than they're hitting other communities," said Richard Besser, president and chief executive officer of the Robert Wood Johnson Foundation (RWJF).

Culture of Health in Practice, Alonzo L. Plough. Oxford University Press (2020) © Robert Wood Johnson Foundation
DOI: 10.1093/oso/9780190071400.001.0001

A key component of building a Culture of Health in America is really ensuring that communities are becoming resilient, that they have what it takes to withstand both the everyday threats to health as well as the disasters that are becoming more and more common. —Richard Besser

This chapter opens with a summary of recent studies on the impact and health consequences of climate change. Elizabeth Yeampierre then explains how social injustice and climate change intersect. She makes a powerful argument that indigenous people, people of color, and low-income communities—in short, the front-line communities—have a voice in developing solutions and must be central to any effort that addresses disparities created by climate change.

Liesel Ritchie provides an in-depth review of environmental stressors associated with technological disasters—events caused by human error—and their impact from a sociological perspective. Ritchie and Yeampierre conclude with a portrait of resilience, focusing on the citizens of a Gulf Research Program, residents of Sunset Park in Brooklyn, and the citizens of Puerto Rico, whose efforts are described in a Spotlight profile.

The Evidence and Urgency to Address Climate Change

At the end of 2018, two well-publicized scientific reports described what the Earth will look like in the throes of continued global warming and climate change.

"A Deafening, Piercing Smoke Alarm"

The United Nations Intergovernmental Panel on Climate Change (IPCC) reported in October 2018 that world leaders had less than 12 years to act to reduce carbon emissions before efforts to hold warming to moderate levels were certain to fail.[3] The UN scientists cautioned that nations around the world needed to take "unprecedented" actions to cut their carbon emissions over the next decade.[4]

"What we've done is said what the world needs to do," said Jim Skea, co-chair of the IPCC Panel, the UN body for assessing the science related to climate change. "It's now their responsibility to decide whether they can act on it."[5]

[The IPCC report is] like a deafening, piercing smoke alarm going off in the kitchen. We have to put out the fire.—Erik Solheim, executive director, UN Environment Program[6]

This landmark report by a leading nonpartisan, scientific body prompted two congressional lawmakers to introduce a far-reaching legislative measure known as the "Green New Deal" to remake the U.S. economy and eliminate all U.S. carbon emissions by 2025.[7] The *New York Times* noted that the plan, a long way from being approved or adopted, "has had a rocky start, but it has also changed the national conversation. That alone is reason to applaud it."

"A Severe Threat to America's Health:" The National Climate Assessment Report

Released in November 2018, the fourth National Climate Assessment report warned of interconnected, cascading health risks caused by climate change if nothing is done to curtail greenhouse gas emission. The authors foreshadow America's declining crops, a surge of tropical diseases such as dengue fever, a shortage of drinkable water, and tens of millions of people exposed to extreme heat.[8,9]

> *Climate change creates new risks and exacerbates existing vulnerabilities in communities across the United States, presenting growing challenges to human health and safety, quality of life, and the rate of economic growth. — National Climate Assessment report[10]*

The report included "an unmistakable message," according to one news analysis: "The effects of climate change—including deadly wildfires, increasingly debilitating hurricanes, and heat waves—are already battering the United States, and the danger of more such catastrophes is worsening. The report's authors say they are more certain than ever that climate change poses a severe threat to Americans' health and pocketbooks, as well as to the country's infrastructure and natural resources."[11]

Produced by 13 federal departments and agencies and overseen by the U.S. Global Change Research Program, the National Climate Assessment report provided critical findings in 12 categories often highlighted as part of a Culture of Health. Here are summary highlights from three of them—communities, health, and indigenous peoples:[12]

- **Communities:** Climate change has created new health and economic risks and "exacerbates existing vulnerabilities in communities across the United States." The impacts within and across regions will not be distributed equally.
  - "People who are already vulnerable, including lower-income and other marginalized communities, have lower capacity to prepare for and cope

with extreme weather and climate-related events and are expected to experience greater impacts."

- **Health:** Impacts from climate change increasingly threaten the health and well-being of the American people, particularly disenfranchised and vulnerable populations.
  - "Changes in temperature and precipitation are increasing air quality and health risks from wildfire and ground-level ozone pollution. Rising air and water temperatures and more intense extreme events are expected to increase exposure to waterborne and foodborne diseases, affecting food and water safety. . . . The frequency and severity of allergic illnesses, including asthma and hay fever, are expected to increase as a result of a changing climate."
  - "Climate change is also projected to alter the geographic range and distribution of disease-carrying insects and pests, exposing more people to ticks that carry Lyme disease and mosquitoes that transmit viruses such as Zika, West Nile, and dengue, with varying impacts across the regions. Communities in the Southeast, for example, are particularly vulnerable to the combined health impacts from vector-borne disease, heat, and flooding."
  - In 2017, 157 million more people were exposed to heat-related health risks than in 2000; the report found that some of the largest increases in heat-related mortality in future years will occur in the Northeast. Because heat stress not only kills people directly but also leads to kidney and cardiovascular diseases, the report labeled heat stress as "among the biggest threats human face in a warming climate."
- **Indigenous Peoples:** Climate change increasingly threatens the livelihoods, economies, health, and cultural identities of indigenous communities "by disrupting interconnected social, physical, and ecological systems."
  - "Many Indigenous peoples are reliant on natural resources for their economic, cultural, and physical well-being and are often uniquely affected by climate change." The impacts of climate change are expected to increasingly disrupt indigenous peoples' livelihoods (agriculture, forestry, fishing, recreation, tourism); physical and mental health; and cultural and community continuity. "Throughout the United States, climate-related impacts are causing some Indigenous peoples to consider or actively pursue community relocation as an adaptation strategy, presenting challenges associated with maintaining cultural and community continuity."

Global warming is transforming where and how we live and presents growing challenges to human health and quality of life, the economy, and the natural systems that support us. —National Climate Assessment report

The Intersection of Climate Change and Social Justice

The American Public Health Association declared 2017 to be the Year of Climate Change and Health. RWJF also commissioned Climate Central, an independent organization of leading climate change scientists and science journalists, to conduct a landscape assessment of funding and research at the nexus of health and climate change.[13] When the Climate Central report was issued on August 18, 2017, several key findings emerged: "Protecting vulnerable populations in the context of a changing climate will be key; funding of health and climate change is extremely limited; and basic research is no longer needed to establish the threat of climate change to health."[14]

Exactly one month later, Maria, a Category 5 hurricane, slammed into Puerto Rico, devastating the country and underscoring the urgency of the Climate Central findings. With more than 3,000 fatalities and over $100 billion in damages eventually reported, it was the worst natural disaster on record in Puerto Rico and the surrounding islands.[15]

For attorney and activist Elizabeth Yeampierre, the story of what happened in her native Puerto Rico is just one more example of how populations enduring a history of austerity and neglect are most likely to face environmental stressors. In her work to elevate the intersection of climate change and social justice for communities most at risk, she goes beyond messages of resilience in the wake of disaster.

> *It is not just important to talk about resilience but to include resistance, prevention, and a just transition. And a just transition means that those impacted the most speak for themselves and lead the way for change. All the science in the world won't matter without just relationships. —Elizabeth Yeampierre*

The Climate Justice Movement

Yeampierre is the co-chair of the Climate Justice Alliance, a collaborative of more than 68 organizations uniting front-line communities most impacted by climate change. She is also the executive director of UPROSE, Brooklyn's oldest Latino community-based organization. Although she is a community activist trained to listen to all sides, Yeampierre says she is no longer willing to engage with those who do not think climate change is real.

"If you're not thinking about how climate change is going to affect you and the delivery of services around you, then you are not paying attention to the fact that there are wildfires in California, that there was a hurricane in Houston and in Miami, that Hurricane Maria devastated Puerto Rico," she said. "The planet is basically telling you that climate change is here."

Yeampierre focuses on giving a voice to people who are most impacted by climate change, and the advocacy work at UPROSE is done in the interest of what she calls "a just transition." This means moving away from the extraction economy that she says has discriminated against vulnerable populations and moving toward climate solutions led by front-line communities.

> *Those of us who are descendants of colonization and slavery, those of us who have had to deal with the extraction of our land and our labor, we are the ones who are going to be impacted the most by climate change. And we are the ones least responsible for creating it. —Elizabeth Yeampierre*

As one example, she cited the impact of hurricanes and rising water levels on chemical storage in vulnerable areas. Puerto Rico has 23 Superfund sites, and many exploded when Hurricane Maria hit, contaminating water, soil, and air. "How do 23 Superfunds end up on a tiny island like that?" asked Yeampierre, somewhat rhetorically. "That is the history of extraction, of Puerto Rico being the oldest colony in the world, and the fact that things can be done in places where our people live that you can't do in other places. The fact that 23 Superfunds can be on this tiny, tiny, tiny island tells the story of extraction, abuse, toxic exposure, and how corporate America has treated disenfranchised communities."

At the request of Puerto Rican farmers taking recovery into their own hands, UPROSE and Climate Justice Alliance provided support through a people-to-people, just recovery effort (see "Spotlight: A Just Recovery for Puerto Rico").

> *I saw devastation but I didn't see despair. A "just recovery" means Puerto Ricans speak for themselves and own the infrastructure. —Elizabeth Yeampierre*

The First Responders and the Busybody: A Just Recovery in Action

A bit closer to home, another fight for a just recovery is taking place in the Brooklyn neighborhood of Sunset Park. During Superstorm Sandy in the fall of 2012, the industrial sector of the waterfront community was heavily impacted by millions of gallons of water. Sunset Park also sustained extreme wind damage that uprooted trees and caused substantial damage to property and lives throughout the area. Two months after the storm, UPROSE hosted a community meeting in Sunset Park to engage with community members. "We are the first responders!" declared the local people, who immediately jumped in with community resilience strategies and plans for organizing themselves to address the problems.[16]

"We know that in a community, the first responder is that busybody who's always looking out the window, who knows everybody's business. That person knows who's on dialysis, who has diabetes, who's hooking up with whom. Those are the people who are your first responders," said Yeampierre.

"They need to be empowered and provided with the resources to lead," she continued, with passion and urgency. "And if they're not, we will fail. Because it doesn't matter that we've got experts who understand what the technology should look like. It doesn't matter that we can measure different levels of contaminants and that we can actually do GIS mapping to show where the vulnerabilities exist. We know how to do all those things. And none of that will matter unless we build just relationships, unless we engage in a process of self-transformation and agree that privilege must be checked."

> *And that means that solutions are local. That people cannot helicopter into our community with the solutions. That you have to be able to complement what we're doing—not supplant local leadership and not compete with us in a time of crisis. —Elizabeth Yeampierre*

Warned Yeampierre, "What is coming our way is going to take out the most vulnerable. If we believe in justice, if we believe that climate change is here, and if we care about public health and how that affects children and our elderly, then we need to be able to support intergenerational front-line leadership. The people impacted the most are that front line. We need the folks who believe in justice and have a commitment to antiracism to support us in doing that."

Corrosive Communities, White Noise, and Environmental Stressors

Liesel Ashley Ritchie is the first to admit that her academic and research career is based on a series of "unfortunate opportunities." Her story begins with one of them: the 1989 *Exxon Valdez* oil spill, one of the worst human-caused environmental disasters in this country's history.

While working on her PhD at Mississippi State University in 2001, Ritchie joined a research team that had been studying the impacts of the *Exxon Valdez* oil spill since it happened. The spill took place northwest of Cordova, Alaska—a commercial fishing community of 2,500 people with a subsistence heritage rooted in Alaska Native culture. There, an oil tanker ran aground on a well-marked reef, sending somewhere between 11 and 33 million gallons of crude oil (estimates vary widely) into Alaska's Prince William Sound and causing an environmental disaster that upended the entire area's fishing economy and transformed the local ecology.

In a book called *Crime and Criminal Justice in Disaster,* Ritchie and co-authors Duane A. Gill and J. Steven Picou described the Cordova event in a chapter about technological disasters:[17]

> *After two calm days during which the spill could have been contained, a powerful storm spread the oil beyond control. As a result, more than 27,000 square miles, including 1,180 miles of Alaskan coastline, were oiled. The destruction of habitat, fish, marine mammals and birds was beyond that for any spill in the history of oil transportation. Initial estimates suggested more than 250,000 birds, 4,400 sea otters, 300 harbor seals, 250 bald eagles, 22 orca whales and countless numbers of fish perished in the immediate aftermath of the spill. However, the inability to accurately document damages caused by the spill suggests these are conservative estimates.*
>
> *The Exxon Valdez oil spill was also devastating to residents of the small Alaska Native villages and commercial fishing communities. These "renewal resource communities" derive their "cultural, social, and economic existence" from the "harvest and use of renewable resources."... Initial social impacts included elevated levels of family conflict, domestic violence, increased consumption of alcohol and drugs, collective trauma, social disruption, economic uncertainty, community strain, and psychological stress.... Alaska Natives and commercial fishermen were the two social groups most negatively affected by initial and long-term impacts of this disaster.*

When Ritchie joined the research team, she recalled, "I was in a position to bring a fresh set of eyes to the table." Initially, her role was to collect data on psycho-social stress, defined as the interaction between social factors and individual thoughts and behaviors. During interviews in the Cordova region, she heard stories of how the community's social capital had declined. "They didn't actually use that term—'social capital'—but they did say, 'Our warriors are tired.' This is a verbatim quote: '*Our warriors are tired.*'"

Translated? Nearly 12 years after the oil spill, cumulative stressors—from ecological disruption and economic hardships to ongoing litigation seeking restitution and community upheaval—played out in the community's ability to respond to challenges. If there was a mud landslide, a snow avalanche, or a boat in distress, the Cordova community could still rally with short bursts of energy to fix an immediate problem. But asked to deal with a local hospital in danger of closing, they were slow to develop a plan of action that required collaborative decision-making and long-term planning.

Said Ritchie, "They started telling me, 'We just don't have the energy and the wherewithal at this point to do things collectively that were to the advantage of the community.' There was too much conflict in the community. Neighbors didn't get along as well as they had. Family members were sort of pitted against family members in terms of whether they made money off of working on the cleanup from the spill, or whether they were shut out of contracts and work."

> *It was very low-lying. But it was this constant, underlying white noise of what we call "a corrosive community."*—Liesel Ritchie

The Unique Impact of Technological Disasters

In May 2004, Ritchie finished her dissertation, "Voices of Cordova: Social Capital in the Wake of the *Exxon Valdez* Oil Spill." In a series of academic positions that followed at the University of Colorado Boulder, she continued to focus on the social impacts of technological disasters. These are typically institutional failures in which people or entities fail to do what they are supposed to do "to look out for the good of humankind," said Ritchie.

Other technological disasters include the dumping of toxic wastes at Love Canal (New York, 1978); the near meltdown of the nuclear plant at Three-Mile Island (Pennsylvania, 1979); the industrial gas leak tragedy in Bhopal (India, 1984); the catastrophic nuclear accident at Chernobyl (Ukraine, 1986); the Tennessee Valley Authority (TVA) coal ash spill (Tennessee, 2008); the BP Deepwater Horizon Oil Spill (Gulf of Mexico, 2010); and the lead water crisis in Flint (Michigan, 2015).

> *We are facing what Kai Erickson [an American sociologist] has referred to as a "new species of trouble" that "scare human beings in new and special ways . . . and elicit an uncanny fear in us."* —Liesel Ritchie

With funding from the National Science Foundation, Ritchie studied three of these disasters extensively: the *Exxon Valdez* oil spill, the TVA coal ash spill, and the BP Deepwater Horizon oil spill. Ritchie documented a "corrosive community" phenomenon that is unique to these kinds of events. She explained why: "When you look at something like a tornado, which is strictly an act of god, so to speak, everyone is kind of in the same boat. In natural disasters, we more commonly see what we call a 'therapeutic community,' where individuals come together and are able to rally around each other because they're in the same situation. At the other end of the spectrum is a corrosive community, where you have these technological disasters where there's actually a party to blame, someone who was responsible for the event as well as the clean-up and compensation for damages. And there are all sorts of winners and losers in those cases."

Ritchie has identified sources of the resulting psychological stress, frustration, and social and physical anxiety, including:

- **Contested interpretations.** Ritchie said there are always several ways to understand these disasters, and often "it depends on whose science it is—whether it is the industry science, government science, or independent science. Contested interpretations are difficult for everyone." Contested science does "little to alleviate uncertainty," she said. "These elevated concerns feed into intrusive stress and avoidance behaviors."[18]

  In her 2018 study on resource loss (loss of life, injury, damage to or loss of property) and psychosocial stress following the TVA coal ash spill, Ritchie documented how "an inability to locate reliable information about potential short- and long-term health effects, uncertainty about the extent of environmental damage, fear of plummeting property values, and uncertain implications for community stability created an atmosphere of confusion among area residents."

  The strongest contributors to this spill-related stress were lost resources, or the threat of their loss, as well as increased perceptions of risk connected to experiences with the spill; beliefs about economic and environmental impacts; concerns about health; and perceived social disruption. The coal ash spill, she wrote, "has given rise to a classic 'contested science' scenario and competing environmental and public health narratives."[19]

- **Invisible trauma.** With every environmental event, there are psychological effects and consequences that are difficult to see or track, a phenomenon labeled "invisible trauma" in the late 1980s by anthropologist and physician Henry Vyner. "One of the primary concerns regarding environmental impacts and how these impacts ultimately affect communities and groups has to do with ecological damage that is difficult to detect," Ritchie wrote in an article called "The BP Disaster as an *Exxon Valdez* Rerun." "Even more challenging is assessing damage that may not emerge until years after initial contamination."[20]

  In their analyses of the BP oil spill, explained Ritchie, "there were scientists on the same team who couldn't agree on how extensive the damage was and how long the damage might be in play in the Gulf of Mexico. Some said it could take up to 20 years, others said it would be healed much more quickly than that. They just couldn't agree."

- **Cultural vulnerability and long-term adverse health outcomes.** A community's strength can also be its vulnerability, particularly after an environmental disaster that is innately connected to a community's livelihood and generations of customs and traditions. Impacted communities experience a loss of control and increased vulnerability, resulting in anxiety, uncertainty, social disruption, conflict, and psychological stress.

    Because the long-term adverse health outcomes of toxic exposures can unfold slowly, communities often struggle to find closure, creating a host of other chronic challenges.

    In her studies, Ritchie found that the uncertain ecological and economic impacts associated with environmental disasters also can foster lingering health issues. A comparative study of the Valdez and BP oil spills revealed similar social and psychological impacts, with elevated levels of stress in both communities.[21]

    Ritchie explained that indigenous peoples in Canada and the United States are particularly at risk. "These groups are dependent on renewable natural resources such as marine life and other kinds of environmental resources, which makes them much more vulnerable to the hazards, disasters, and results of toxic environmental contamination. Some of the First Nations peoples, some of the Alaska natives, some of the Native Americans—they have been very resilient until these kinds of activities come into play in our culture and society."

[Environmental disasters and associated stressors] can ruin livelihoods, ruin sociocultural activities. This can go on for generations and damage the way people have traditionally lived for thousands of years. This is not environmental justice.—Liesel Ritchie

- **Secondary trauma from post-event bureaucracy.** Ritchie found that the litigation and claims processing that often follow technological disasters create a "pressure cooker effect," leading once-supportive social interactions to become sources of stress that adversely affect the whole community. For instance, Ritchie's data showed that although only 10 percent of the survey respondents were involved in the BP Deepwater Horizon compensation processes, nearly 66 percent of all respondents indicated that the processes were as distressing as the oil spill itself.[22]

    A lack of consistency and transparency, she wrote after the *Exxon Valdez* spill, "contributes to a corrosive community by reducing trust, weakening social connections and networks, altering social discourse, diminishing feelings of goodwill, and violating norms of reciprocity."[23]

At the same time, the slow and uneven legal process makes it virtually impossible for those affected to fully move on with their lives. Damage claims in the Exxon case were not definitively settled for more than 20 years. And when the Supreme Court voted in 2008 to reduce the plaintiffs' original $2.5 billion punitive damage award to $507 million, it was another blow to a damaged community. Wrote Ritchie: "Perceptions of recreancy became embedded in the collective conscious of Cordova and contributed to an apathy that adversely affected perceptions of and relationships with big business, government and the judicial system."[24]

Twenty-five years after the *Valdez* ran aground, Ritchie reported that Cordova was moving toward recovery from spill-related mental health impacts, but that "former litigants and Alaska Natives continued to be at higher risk" of psychological problems. And the chronic ecological impacts of the disaster continued to unfold. Only 10 of the 26 species impacted have recovered. Tragically, for a community that so depended on it, the herring fishery is not among them.[25]

> From traditional Native villages to communities like Cordova, the early spring return of herring had held spiritual and symbolic meanings, in addition to being an economic resource. Whereas Cordova's fishing season used to begin in March, it now begins in May with king and red salmon. The resulting sociocultural changes may be permanent. —Liesel Ritchie

Getting on the Other Side of the Disaster

After decades spent studying technological disasters, Ritchie well understood the importance of resilience and decided to shift her focus to what she called, "getting on the other side of the disaster." Said Ritchie, "If we could explain to people what they might be facing if something goes wrong when one of the projects in oil and gas development comes through, then we have an opportunity to actually build that in on the front end."

> We may or may not be able to prevent the disaster. We may or may not be able to avoid the hazard. But perhaps we can do something on the front end that would help to mitigate these kinds of disaster effects from a social impact perspective. —Liesel Ritchie

Experts in business, science, health, and philanthropy are now increasingly focused on strengthening a community's ability to withstand environmental events. Both Ritchie and Yeampierre provided examples of this movement.

The Gulf Research Program: Nurturing Resilience Before a Crisis

Ritchie, now associate director at the Center for the Study of Disasters and Extreme Events at Oklahoma State University, serves on the advisory board of the Gulf Research Program, established in 2013 through the BP oil spill settlement.[26] Based within the National Academies of Sciences, Engineering, and Medicine, the program looks to catalyze advances in science, practice, and capacity to generate long-term benefits for the Gulf of Mexico region and the nation, more broadly.

One of the four initiatives that help operationalize the mission of the Gulf Research Program is known as Thriving Communities; social justice is at its core. Instead of focusing on infrastructure needs or the built environment, the program supports the study of the human dynamics—such as physical and mental health, social cohesiveness, and social and economic well-being—that influence a community's ability to cope. Recent grant awards have addressed the science and practice of resilience in the coastal communities of the Gulf of Mexico, and documented how environmental stressors impact the livelihood of Louisiana's coastal indigenous communities.[27]

RWJF is collaborating with the Gulf Research Program to jointly support four studies under the Thriving Communities umbrella focused on enhancing the science and practice of community resilience with a focus on health equity.[28] These studies are intended to analyze how "those most directly affected by the conditions on the ground need to play a meaningful role in defining their own problems, designing the interventions intended to solve them, and shaping research questions that test those areas," said Tracy Costigan, RWJF senior program officer, Research–Evaluation–Learning.[29] The projects are based in Louisiana and Alabama.[30]

Resilience Preparation in Sunset Park

At UPROSE, Yeampierre pointed to three Sunset Park campaigns specifically focused on resilience preparation.

- **The Sunset Park Climate Justice Center.** In the wake of Superstorm Sandy, the community urged UPROSE to help organize them to prepare for the next crisis and put the neighborhood on a path to sustainability, adaptation, and resilience. In response, UPROSE launched the Sunset Park Climate Justice Center, New York City's first grassroots-led climate adaptation and community resiliency planning project. Key goals include:

- Building the capacity of Sunset Park's leaders and local businesses to respond effectively to severe weather events, coordinate the allocation of community resources, and mitigate the impacts of future environmental stressors, including the release of harmful chemicals.
- Developing tools and partnerships to transition the Sunset Park industrial area from a traditional 20th-century model into a 21st-century climate-resilient and sustainable area. According to UPROSE, "Such a transition will ensure the long-term availability of business development and employment opportunities for NYC's largest walk-to-work community, Sunset Park."
- Engaging community members and local businesses in leadership development and in a block-by-block, building-by-building process to assess, map, and build relationships that foster a bottom-up response to climate change.
- **The Sunset Park Green Resilient Improvement District (GRID).** The Sunset Park GRID is an association of small merchants facing the greatest environmental and economic risks. Through GRID, which is dedicated to the dual goals of revitalization and resilience, UPROSE has "conducted research, recruitment, education, and leadership development for businesses" to increase their chances for "environmental and economic survival."
- **Grassroots Research to Action in Sunset Park (GRASP).** As part of the Climate Justice Center, UPROSE formed GRASP to study hazardous chemicals along the Sunset Park waterfront. With funding from the National Institute of Environmental Health Sciences, GRASP is conducting a five-year project to work closely with small businesses—particularly local auto shops—to reduce the risk of chemical releases during extreme weather events.[31]

All of these efforts and others give Yeampierre hope. "My mom always said when I was little, 'You can't cover the sky with your hand.' What she meant is, you have to see the whole sky. And so I *see* it. I *see* the threats and I *see* the challenges. And every day I work because climate change is here. I work hard every single day, and I'm not alone in doing that."

I'm part of what is a leaderful community that is made up mostly of front-line people of color, working with each other in a way that makes it possible for each of us to be stronger in our own community. That makes me happy. That gives me hope. That makes me feel like, "We got this." And that warms my heart. —Elizabeth Yeampierre

A Final Word

Nearly six months after three catastrophic hurricanes devastated diverse areas of the United States, RWJF in March 2018 launched an initiative called Integrative Action for Resilience. Designed to help communities prepare for, withstand, and recover from disasters, the initiative seeks to foster partnership between communities and researchers. Four projects were selected: building community leadership and civic infrastructure to improve resilience in Miami–Dade County, Florida, and to produce findings that help communities nationwide; developing a practical model for a climate-resilient community in East Boston, Mass., to enhance preparedness; evaluating the impact of a cross-sector community collaboration that addresses trauma, police-community relations, and community resilience in Jackson, Miss; and developing a strong cadre of intergenerational citizen leaders to advance resilience and equity in North Montgomery County, Miss. "We urgently need to understand the confluence of factors that helps American communities develop resilience," noted Costigan.[32]

Also, through its Health and Climate Solutions program, which launched in 2018, the Foundation solicited proposals for assessments of community-based approaches that address climate adaptation or mitigation, while improving health and well-being. The funded projects have implemented equity-focused approaches for at least one year that direct attention to one or more determinants of health—including but not limited to food systems, access to water, and housing.[33]

"One thing is clear from these efforts: tackling the effect of climate change requires that leaders from all sectors work together. That includes health care, public health, community development, housing, urban design, environmental safety, business and more," said RWJF's Alonzo L. Plough, PhD, MPH, MA, chief science officer and vice president, Research–Evaluation–Learning.[34]

> *When we can find ways to address climate change alongside other sectors, we can expect better health, stronger communities, and greater equity in health and well-being. That's a triple win. —Alonzo L. Plough*

Chapter 9 Spotlight: A Just Recovery
for Puerto Rico

Just two months after Hurricane Maria hit Puerto Rico in September 2017, Elizabeth Yeampierre returned to the home of her ancestors. "I went with a really heavy heart," she said of her return to Puerto Rico. "My heart literally hurt."

The devastation was excruciating to see—neighborhoods completely destroyed, the grief of widespread death, the struggle to clear the wreckage and rebuild without electricity, food, running water, or supplies. "It was like a chapter out of Octavia Butler's Parable of the Sower," *she said, referencing the science fiction novel set in the 2020s, when society has largely collapsed due to climate change, growing wealth inequality, and corporate greed.*

But Yeampierre also saw scenes that "gave me tremendous hope. What I found were children in Orocovis who were farming, showing up at the farm two days after the storm because they were going to try and harvest food for their family. I found these anchors all over the island where people were sharing food."

Yeampierre had returned to Puerto Rico after the hurricane as part of the national Our Power PR initiative,[1] launched by the Climate Justice Alliance, UPROSE, Grassroots International, Greenpeace, and other organizations with a goal to engage with Puerto Ricans in a people-to-people just recovery.

As defined by the climate justice movement, a "just recovery" is one led by the people most impacted, rather than by far-reaching government initiatives or exploitative developers who rush in to capitalize on an extremely vulnerable population. The term first surfaced after Hurricane Harvey devastated Houston in August 2017, a month before Hurricane Maria hit Puerto Rico.

Yeampierre and author Naomi Klein embraced the term several months later when they wrote that a just recovery in Puerto Rico "is a Puerto Rican recovery designed by Puerto Ricans."[2]

During her September visit, Yeampierre met at the University of Puerto Rico with 60 organizations from around the island to put together the Our Power PR platform to address food and economic sovereignty and support Puerto Ricans in control of their own recovery.

Two early examples of this platform:

- *Organización Boricuá, the Our Power PR partner on the island, helped distribute solar-powered generators and increased their agroecological work in an* effort to support self-reliant communities that no longer depend on traditional power sources or food. Before the hurricane, Puerto Rico received 98 percent of its power from fossil fuels and 85 percent of that from the United States.

- Efforts to revive local agriculture through local farmers who moved to embrace the methods of agroecology, an approach that taps both indigenous knowledge of food production and modern technology. The farmers and the Our Power PR campaign advocated for more community-controlled agricultural cooperatives, and groups known as "agroecology brigades" traveled around the island to deliver seeds and soil to communities.

In January 2018, the Our Power PR campaign announced other demands: justice under the Jones Act, the shipping law that requires all goods entering Puerto Rio from the mainland to arrive via U.S. ships, driving up costs and limiting delivery options; the end of PROMESA, a 2016 federal law that restructured Puerto Rico's nearly $74 billion debt; a robust federal aid package to support a just recovery; and support for brigades and donations to grassroots groups on the ground.[3]

Efforts to drive a just recovery continue today. Representatives from Our Power PR regularly travel to Puerto Rico to work with Organización Boricuá, meeting with agroecologists and members of the labor movement who support local communities taking charge of their own recovery.[4]

On September 20, 2018, the one-year anniversary of Hurricane Maria's landfall in Puerto Rico, Yeampierre stood in solidarity with hundreds of political leaders, artists, citizens, and activists in New York City's Union Square to remind the world that Puerto Ricans are still fighting "to remain, reclaim, and rebuild." With the Puerto Rican flag held high, Yeampierre's message rang out over the park:[5]

> Hurricane Maria landed on a legacy of austerity, neglect, and colonialism in Puerto Rico and opened the floodgates to those who prosper on the pain and loss of people of color—those responsible for climate change. Climate Justice is the resistance to a history of extraction of land and labor in the Global South. We know this is a fight for our survival. And we are ready.

The Green Health Care Revolution

*Kathy Gerwig, Vice President, Employee Safety, Health, and Wellness, and
Environmental Stewardship Officer, Kaiser Permanente*

In 1996, the U.S. Environmental Protection Agency (EPA) reported that the health care sector was one of the largest environmental polluters on the planet, operating thousands of medical waste incinerators that released mercury, dioxin, and other toxic chemicals into the air every day. According to one estimate at the time, hospitals produced more than 5.9 million tons of waste each year—the equivalent of 33 pounds per hospital bed.[1]

The irony was lost on no one. The sector committed to healing was a major polluter.

In the two decades since the EPA's announcement, the health care industry has worked steadily to embrace environmental stewardship and make system-wide changes to decrease its considerable environmental footprint. As anchor institutions in their communities, hospitals and health care systems are in a unique position to do this: they have the resources, the authority, and the responsibility to lead by example and to reduce the health hazards that literally bring patients to their door.

What many now call the green health care revolution is a "lesson of hope," believes Kathy Gerwig, environmental stewardship officer for Kaiser Permanente, the country's largest not-for-profit health plan and a leading integrated health care system. In her book *Greening Health Care: How Hospitals Can Heal the Planet*, she wrote, "The future of health care holds a promise of planetary healing that extends far beyond the system of health care."[2]

This chapter describes the green health care revolution, a movement that includes efforts to: reduce greenhouse gas emissions; reduce toxic chemicals and materials in hospital buildings and operating rooms; streamline and improve supply chains; reduce material, water, and energy waste; foster farm-to-table food options; enhance green investment opportunities; and improve waste disposal practices. It traces the evolution of the movement since 1996 and the

Culture of Health in Practice, Alonzo L. Plough. Oxford University Press (2020) © Robert Wood Johnson Foundation
DOI: 10.1093/oso/9780190071400.001.0001

founding of Health Care Without Harm (HCWH), an organization created to help health care systems chart a new path forward in response to the EPA's announcement. Gerwig describes how and why Kaiser Permanente, in concert with Health Care Without Harm, emerged as a health care systems leader in efforts to promote a myriad of greening health care initiatives and to decrease its carbon footprint.[3] (The carbon footprint is defined as a measurement of carbon dioxide and other greenhouse gas emissions created through power resources and materials bought and used, taking into account the life span of materials long after they have left the possession of an organization or individual.)

Granted, the challenge remains daunting. An estimated 10 percent of harmful U.S. emissions still originate from health systems, making them significant contributors to the problem of climate change.[4] According to a recent study, the U.S. health care sector would be the world's 13th-largest emitter of greenhouse gases if it were ranked as a nation.[5]

> *We are a big contributor and we should be a big part of solving the problem. Hospitals are obligated to meet community health needs. What bigger need do we have today than the existential threat of climate change? —Kathy Gerwig*

The Revolution Begins

In many ways, the green health care revolution began in the summer of 1996 when Kathy Gerwig met Gary Cohen at an environmental conference at Tufts University outside Boston, Mass.

A former environmental and economic development consultant, Gerwig had joined Kaiser Permanente three years earlier to help develop its environmental stewardship strategies. Cohen, a committed environmental activist, had worked on behalf of the survivors of the 1984 Union Carbide pesticide plant explosion in Bhopal, India, an event that inspired his focus on the growing dangers of toxic chemicals. From there, he shifted to examining health care systems and their lack of environmental sustainability and stewardship.[6]

Cohen had called Gerwig before the Tufts event to explain his plans to form the advocacy organization that became Health Care Without Harm, dedicated to cleaning up and limiting the use of toxic materials in the health care sector. He was forming the group with Charlotte Brody, a registered nurse who shared his concern about the routine burning of thousands of tons of chlorine-based plastic medical waste and trash at an estimated 5,000 onsite or remote incinerators around the country.

As described in her book, Gerwig confessed to some trepidation. "As a representative of the nation's largest non-profit health care organization—and an industry known for caution and risk aversion in the face of major change—I did not know what to expect from this activist," she wrote. "Would I be viewed as the enemy, an unwitting agent of the chemical industry?"

Gerwig soon discovered that Cohen and Brody's strategy was "not to blame the health care industry for its ways," she wrote. "They were more interested in collaboration than confrontation, in working with partners rather than battling enemies."

Brody explained their perspective: "Setting up the good-guy activists against the evil bad-guy hospitals creates a dynamic where real change is hardly possible. And even if you do get some change, it doesn't create a trajectory of hope. Instead, if we create a dialogue among participants, all of whom have strengths and weaknesses, you can get much farther faster."

Gerwig left their first meeting thinking she had established some valuable contacts, but she did not yet realize how transformative this relationship would be. Cohen, however, already had an inkling.

"I remember going back to my colleagues and telling them that I thought Kaiser Permanente was going to be a partner with us," he said. "It was like picking a lottery ticket from the ground and it turns out to be the winning number."

A Greening Health Care Alliance Takes Shape

One of the first issues that demanded Gerwig's attention was the ubiquitous use of polyvinyl chloride (PVC, a leading source of dioxin pollution) in hospitals in everything from intravenous tubing, blood bags, exam gloves, and feeding tubes to furniture and vinyl floors. Particularly devastating to Gerwig was the use of PVC in neonatal intensive care units, and the horror of one neonatal nurse manager when she learned that PVC plastic products contained the toxic chemical DEHP (di2-ethylhexyl phthalate) to make them soft and flexible, and that this chemical plasticizer was leaching into the solutions used to treat her newborn patients.

> *The very equipment we were using to support life for these critically ill and preterm infants was capable of leaching a potentially toxic substance into their bodies that could result in reproductive abnormalities over a lifetime.* —Kathy Gerwig

As Gerwig explained in her book: "PVC is one of the many disturbing examples of the paradox of health care's role in environmental pollution. In the course of providing health care to individuals, we are inadvertently using chemicals and materials that are hazardous to human health. We generate pollution and wastes that become environmental contributors to disease. Institutions dedicated to human health were among the primary culprits in poisoning the atmosphere with toxic emissions that, at even low levels, were contributing to human cancers and infertility. The fact that laws and regulations required incineration of many pathology and chemical wastes only made the irony more painful."[7]

Health Care Without Harm was born out of this paradox, Gerwig reasoned. Cohen agreed.

"Health care is one of the only sectors of the entire economy that has an ethical framework as a centerpiece of its profession. Caregivers take an oath to 'first, do no harm,'" said Cohen. "But if you're running a hospital on energy that comes from a coal-fired plant, you are contributing to the asthma rate. If you have a McDonald's restaurant in the lobby of your hospital, you may be contributing to the rampant obesity rate and all the health and environmental problems associated with that. If I'm a hospital leader, I want to model for others to do the right thing from a disease prevention standpoint."[8]

In June 1998, the American Hospital Association and the EPA signed a landmark agreement to advance pollution prevention efforts in health care facilities around the nation.[9] And in 1999, Kaiser Permanente became an official member of Health Care Without Harm in order to petition the U.S. Food and Drug Administration (FDA) to require manufacturers to label plastic products that could expose patients to DEHP. The petition was rejected—but the unbreakable alliance between Kaiser Permanente and Health Care Without Harm would prove to be "transformative for both of us," according to Gerwig.

"In many ways, our two organizations, along with several other mission-driven hospital systems that joined the movement early on, were embarking on a long and ongoing journey," Gerwig wrote.

> Our journey would take those early concerns about environmental health and its links to human health from the fringes of the nation's health care industry to its mainstream. —Kathy Gerwig[10]

When other health care organizations began to approach Gerwig for advice and information about how to start environmentally safe programs at their own medical centers, she gave a terse, but unequivocal answer: "Your first stop is Health Care Without Harm."

Success Stories from Health Care Without Harm

For two decades, Health Care Without Harm has worked to inform and influence major health systems, health ministries, health care workers, medical device manufacturers, group purchasing organizations, and environmental policy.

It has grown into a broad-based international coalition of hundreds of organizations in 55 countries, with offices in the United States, Europe, and Asia.

A MacArthur Foundation Fellows Award winner, Cohen is also president and co-founder of Practice Greenhealth, a nonprofit membership organization within Health Care Without Harm that was developed with support from the Robert Wood Johnson Foundation (RWJF).[11] Practice Greenhealth now has over 1,200 members ranging from health care organizations to suppliers who are dedicated to creating safer, sustainable workplaces and improving the health of their patients, staff, and communities.

What a Greening Health Care Movement Looks Like

Health Care Without Harm (HCWH) presents environmental impact stories on its website, stories that help illustrate why Gerwig encourages everyone to make the organization their first stop along the greening health care movement:[12]

- **Climate change and public health:** HCWH has played a leading role in rebranding climate change as the greatest public health threat and building a global coalition of health care systems and leaders to create a low-carbon society and advocate for sensible policies to accelerate the transition away from fossil fuels.
- **Medical waste:** More than 4,500 medical waste incinerators have closed in the United States, and hundreds more have closed across Europe, with many hospitals switching to safer and more cost-effective nonburning waste treatment technologies.
- **Medical waste in vaccination programs:** HCWH partnered with the Philippine Department of Health in 2004 to provide measles vaccines to 18 million children and safely dispose of vaccination syringes without burning them.
- **Mercury:** Almost all U.S. hospitals and all major pharmacies have switched to safer nonmercury thermometers. The European Union has banned both mercury thermometers and blood pressure devices that use mercury. An international treaty called the Minamata Convention on Mercury calls for the phasing out of mercury-based measuring devices in global production and use by 2020.
- **Environmentally preferable purchasing:** The top group-purchasing organizations in the United States—representing more than 70 percent of buying power for the nation's health care industry—have committed to taking mercury products off contract, and to listing DEHP-free/PVC-free medical devices in catalogues. HCWH created large-scale demand in health care for furnishings that do not contain brominated flame retardants, and is educating

its 1,200 hospital members about environmentally preferable purchasing. In 2016, HCWH launched its own purchasing cooperative, called Greenhealth Exchange, with nine leading U.S. health care systems.

- **Toxic chemicals and plastics:** Major hospital systems are phasing out PVC medical devices following widespread warnings that harmful phthalates leach out of them. The health care industry's demand for nontoxic products has driven the innovation of PVC-free flooring and wall protection products, and lowered the price of latex-free, vinyl-free nitrile gloves. More than 50 medical societies, cities, and states have passed resolutions to reduce PVC, dioxin, mercury, or medical waste incineration, and there are comparable activities across Europe.
- **Safer chemicals policy:** The European Union passed a major reform of chemicals policy, which will provide health and safety data for thousands of chemicals and help move the market toward safer alternatives. HCWH is working to embed a similar framework into policy and purchasing strategies in the United States and around the world.
- **Healthy food in health care:** HCWH developed a program to transform the food purchasing practices of health care. In the United States, more than 1,200 hospitals are changing their purchasing by supporting farmers' markets on their grounds, buying local and sustainable food, linking healthier food practices with employee and community health, buying antibiotic-free meat, setting up organic farms, running cooking classes, and more. Similar strategies are being deployed by hospitals and health systems all around the world.
- **Green building:** *The Green Guide for Health Care*, developed by HCWH and other partners, is a best-practices guide for health and sustainable building design, construction, and operations for the health care industry. The resource also serves as the foundation for the U.S. Green Building Council's LEED (Leadership in Energy and Environmental Design) for Healthcare. Over 265 major health care projects (representing over 40 million square feet of health care construction) had adopted the guide as their framework as of 2018.

Clearly, efforts at Health Care Without Harm have steadily moved beyond its initial vision "to do less harm." HCWH now promotes a future where the health care sector plays a pivotal role in healing communities and the planet through the concept of restorative health. This vision embraces the construction and operation of facilities that are carbon-neutral, zero-waste, and toxic-free. It also includes helping hospitals leverage their economic and political clout to create both community health and wealth by transforming supply chains and waste streams through purchasing safe products and technologies while modeling and supporting healthy food systems and communities.[13]

*The twenty-first-century hospital can promote the health of its patients, staff,
the general public, and the environment through exercising upstream leverage and downstream influence. —Health Care Without Harm*

Kaiser Permanente: A Greening Health Care Success Story

Kathy Gerwig has helped Kaiser Permanente become a leading example of a
hospital and health care system that sees environmental stewardship as fundamental to its healing role. She began to connect the dots between her environment and health care while growing up in a medical family that lived near West
Virginia's coal mining communities. "I definitely got the connection between
what we see in nature and how that impacts people's health."

This connection was reinforced when her family moved to Santa Barbara
in 1969, around the time of the largest-ever oil spill off the California coast; it
remains the third largest anywhere, after the 1989 *Exxon Valdez* spill and the
2010 Deepwater Horizon spill. "That was another place where I saw the health
consequences to environmental action," said Gerwig, who joined her community for beach cleanups and restoration efforts. The experience made her think
about "how environmental disasters could be avoided in the future through
better environmental policy." (Environmental disasters have both immediate and
enduring consequences for health and community cohesion, a topic explored
in more depth in Chapter 9, "Climate Change, Environmental Stressors, and
Resilience.")

In 1993, Gerwig accepted an offer to be Kaiser Permanente's environmental
stewardship manager, overseeing an operation in eight states and the District of
Columbia. Today, the hospital and health care system serves over 12.3 million
members, has 39 hospitals and 690 medical offices, and is staffed by over 23,000
physicians and more than 200,000 employees, including 59,000 nurses.

Gerwig recognized the challenges right away. "When you think about
hospitals, they operate like small cities," Gerwig explained. "They are 24/7 operations. There's no nighttime power down—it's very energy intensive and it
generates a lot of waste. There's a lot of technology and equipment that is needed
to keep things running and provide health care any time of the day or night. The
business of providing health care is just energy intensive and resource intensive
in every way."

Gerwig always had the backing of her institutional leaders to green the
system. Kaiser Permanente's chairman and chief executive officer Bernard
J. Tyson is recognized as one of the international climate action leaders in global

businesses. And according to Gerwig, environmental stewardship was equally embraced within Kaiser Permanente's board room "because we know that community health is one and the same with patient health." By 2008, she said, "the board put a stake in the ground when we adopted a position statement that said: 'If climate change continues unabated, it will impact our ability to achieve our mission of providing quality, affordable health care to our members and communities.'"

We've had climate action as one of our priority goals in our environmental stewardship program ever since it began over 20 years ago. —Kathy Gerwig

Carbon Neutral in 2020: Kaiser Permanente Makes a Bold Pledge

In 2016, Kaiser Permanente announced an ambitious goal to become carbon neutral in four years. In 2018, Bernard Tyson announced at the Global Climate Action Summit in San Francisco that the health system was definitely on target to meet that goal by the end of 2020. "We believe we can make a difference in the climate and help others to deal with the effects of climate change," Tyson said of the bold pledge.

In *Greening Health Care,* Gerwig described Kaiser Permanente's journey to becoming a leader for positive environmental change, and the products, practices, and principles it has adopted: making food services sustainable, managing hospital waste, greening medical buildings, and buying environmentally responsible products. These are some of the highlights that Gerwig described during the 2018 *Sharing Knowledge* conference, in a subsequent interview, and within her book:

- **Energy:** Kaiser Permanente approaches energy consumption practices from two angles: the demand side (goal: be more efficient) and the supply side (goal: use more renewable and fewer fossil fuel sources).

  - Within its California footprint of 35 hospitals and several hundred medical offices, half of Kaiser Permanente's electricity now comes from renewable sources. "It's very intentional," said Gerwig. Energy use per member has declined 14 percent since 2010; per-member energy costs have declined 18 percent since 2014; and greenhouse gas emissions through Kaiser Permanente fell by 29 percent between 2008 and 2018 —and all of this while membership increased 36 percent.

    We are using a lot more energy than we did in 2008, and yet our greenhouse gas emission footprint is shrinking. Our goal is to be carbon-neutral in 2020. —Kathy Gerwig

- In 2018, Kaiser Permanente reached an agreement to purchase vast amounts of clean energy, a commitment that will fund construction of new utility-scale solar and wind farms, as well as one of the country's largest battery-energy storage systems.[14] With this agreement, Kaiser Permanente will become the largest purchaser of renewable energy in the nation's health care sector.

- Kaiser Permanente has reduced water usage by 14 percent per square foot of building space since 2013. "We want to have a 25 percent reduction by 2025," Gerwig said.

- According to Gerwig, health care organizations spend around $200 billion a year on supplies and nonlabor purchases. Although many of these hospitals have purchasing programs that commit them to buying less harmful chemicals and chemical products, Gerwig noted that Kaiser Permanente has set a stringent standard: By 2025, half of all products they buy will not contain specified toxic chemicals, and they must help meet the organization's waste reduction goals.

  "We need to think about every product that we buy, every supplier we do business with to improve community health in all of those areas at the same time. It can have a huge impact across the economy. What we buy matters, and the supply chain work is really where that lands. And the supply chain is not just for the health care sector—it's the housing, business, and entertainment sectors where it begins to actually turn into trillions of dollars of effort that can make a difference in society overall," said Gerwig.

  I think that's the scale we have to think of if we want to get significantly closer to the aim of a Culture of Health that is truly sustainable and equitable. —Kathy Gerwig

- **Financing and green bonds:** Gerwig pointed out that every health care system has financing and investment portfolios. In 2017, Kaiser Permanente issued $4.4 billion in bonds, $1 billion of which qualified as "green bonds" used to build LEED hospitals, such as the Kaiser Permanente San Diego Medical Center. The San Diego facility is the first LEED Platinum hospital in California. "The green bonds were snapped up like that, and the terms were excellent," said Gerwig. "What that shows us is that there's a hunger by investors who are looking for socially and environmentally responsible investments. That alone can serve as an incentive to build LEED-certified hospitals."

- **Reducing greenhouse gases in operating rooms:** According to Gerwig, halogenated anesthetic gases—the anesthesia used during operations—are some of the most potent greenhouse gases. But "there are plenty of wonderful substitutes for those polluting agents," she said, offering the story as an example of where health care systems can really lean in. "When you engage the chiefs of anesthesiology with the evidence, they want to take action, and that is just what happened in my organization." Between 2014 and 2016, Kaiser Permanente reported a 30 percent reduction in the use of halogenated anesthetic gases. "It made a huge difference in greenhouse gas emission, completely consistent with high-quality, safe, and affordable care."

- **Food for health:** Kaiser Permanente has numerous programs to ensure that food provided in the health care setting is healthy, nutritious, and sustainably sourced.
  - The organization supports more than 55 farmers' markets, which bring local growers directly to medical centers to create healthy food choices, from patient rooms to hospital cafeterias. It has reduced its meat purchasing costs by 18 percent; and by 2025, it aims to buy all of its food locally or from farms and producers that use sustainable practices.[15]
  - Physicians throughout the organization have adopted a "food as medicine" approach to teaching patients that what they eat can have impact on a wide range of diseases, including diabetes, obesity, and heart disease.
  - A new food processing co-op factory being built in the San Francisco East Bay city of Richmond, long considered a food desert, is supported by organizations such as Kaiser Permanente and Health Care Without Harm; it will create 200 new jobs and provide healthy, sustainable food to health care systems, schools, and other consumer organizations. "This collaboration is resulting in an opportunity for community health and wealth that has not existed to date in that very challenged community," Gerwig said.
- **Managing and minimizing hospital wastes:** Like Health Care Without Harm and other health care organizations around the world, Kaiser Permanente emphasizes managing and minimizing hospital wastes. "We're at about a 42 percent recycle rate right now, and we want to have none of our nonhazardous waste going to the landfill by 2025," said Gerwig. Ongoing efforts crisscross the hospital: understanding waste streams, addressing operating room wastes in everything from anesthetic gases to recycling the blue plastic wrap around sterile medical instruments and reprocessing single-use devices, embracing reusable sharps containers, recycling and reusing electronic devices, and recycling construction debris.

One environmental success story especially inspires Gerwig: eliminating toxic intravenous (IV) solution bags. "I am proud to say the IV solution bags purchased by Kaiser Permanente are PVC- and DEHP-free and our IV tubing is DEHP-free," wrote Gerwig, who still thinks often about the nurse who was shocked that equipment once used to care for tiny infants contained chemicals that might do them harm. "The product selection affects nearly 100 tons of medical supplies. As an added bonus, the safe alternative products are saving us close to $5 million a year."

The Green Momentum Goes Mainstream

After two decades, the movement to green the health care industry has garnered widespread enthusiasm, with initiatives surfacing across the country. The following examples reflect how the green momentum continues to go mainstream.

With its 1,200 members, Practice Greenhealth brings together hospitals and health care organizations nationwide to address their health and environmental impacts.[16] In 2014, the Gundersen Health System—headquartered in La Crosse, Wisc., and serving Iowa, Minnesota, and Wisconsin—became the first health system in the nation to offset 100 percent of its energy use with local renewable energy.[17]

At the Global Climate Action Summit in September 2018, Cohen and Gerwig announced the launch of the California Health Care Climate Alliance, comprising five of California's largest health systems, to support climate-smart policies and contribute to the state's ambitious climate goals.[18] Efforts to decarbonize the health care supply chain are also advancing internationally; in November 2018, more than 20 hospitals and health care systems convened the European Healthcare Council to strengthen their commitment to reducing their carbon footprint through "smarter product and pharmaceutical procurements, more sustainable food sourcing, improved packaging, and cleaner forms of transportation."[19]

And last but not least, when *Becker's Healthcare*, a leading source of health care news and analysis, issued its December 2018 list of the "greenest hospitals in America," 68 hospitals were featured, compared with 50 hospitals in 2016. Each one of them pledged to make community environmental stewardship a top priority and embraced projects to reduce waste and energy consumption.[20]

These efforts and many others reinforce Gerwig's optimism about the green health care revolution. "There is a lot of action and momentum today on the part of businesses, local and state governments, civil society, the stakeholders in the communities," she said. "They are showing enormous strength of leadership."

What resonates most is tying climate change directly to individuals, to their community's well-being, to their children's health. There is incredible momentum. And opportunities are right in front of us to act. —Kathy Gerwig

A Final Word

Climate change and pollution disproportionately impact the very young, the poor, the elderly, and those with chronic conditions, making environmental action a fundamental health equity issue. RWJF's commitment to advancing health equity and improving health systems within the context of climate change adaptation has been building for some time. In one such effort, RWJF funded Health Care Without Harm from 2008 to 2012 to identify environmentally sound practices and policies—such as removing harmful toxins and reducing waste—to help health care providers reduce their environmental footprint while protecting the health and safety of their patients and workers.[21] Known now as the Health Care Research Collaborative, that grant brought together some two dozen partners to study opportunities for hospital and health care system executives to make more sustainable choices in health care design, construction, operations, and organization.

RWJF's commitment to transforming health and health care systems "aims to ensure that health care, public health, and social services work together to fully address the goals and needs of the people they serve."[22] When the U.S. Surgeon General issued a "Community Health and Prosperity" Call to Action in late 2018, the response from RWJF President and chief executive officer Richard Besser acknowledged how important private-sector partnerships and environmental health initiatives like those championed by Kaiser Permanente can be in transforming health care systems and creating a Culture of Health that works for everyone.[23]

> *Private-sector businesses are key decision-makers in strategies to improve social and economic factors, health behaviors, and the physical environment.—Richard Besser*

Driving Innovation
Through Medicaid

James B. Becker, MD, Medicaid Medical Director, West Virginia Department of Health and Human Resources

Eliot Fishman, PhD, Senior Director of Policy, Families USA

Ana Fuentevilla, MD, MHCDS, Chief Medical Officer, Optum Population Health Solutions (former Chief Medical Officer, UnitedHealthcare Community & State)

When he signed Medicare and Medicaid into law on the same day—July 30, 1965—President Lyndon B. Johnson changed the trajectory of health care in America. Passed after tumultuous decades of rancor over the role of government in health care, these programs provided nearly universal health insurance for elderly and disabled people and for very low-income families with children.

The Affordable Care Act (ACA), signed by President Barack Obama on March 23, 2010, again after much turmoil, marked another health care milestone. Among its provisions, the ACA opens Medicaid to families with children at somewhat higher income levels than in the past, and for the first time, to low-income nondisabled adults without dependent children, many of whom have significant health risks. As of May 2019, 36 states and the District of Columbia had chosen to expand their Medicaid programs to include these populations.[1]

Medicaid today is a core component of the nation's health care system, providing health coverage to more than 66 million people.[2] One in every five Americans, including one in three children and seven in 10 nursing home residents, receives health insurance through Medicaid.[3] Combined federal and state Medicaid spending totaled $576 billion in federal fiscal year 2017.[4]

With access to millions of people and significant clout over health systems and services, Medicaid is a key resource for promoting health equity. The sheer size of its budget captures the attention of policymakers across the political

Culture of Health in Practice, Alonzo L. Plough. Oxford University Press (2020) © Robert Wood Johnson Foundation
DOI: 10.1093/oso/9780190071400.001.0001

spectrum and at all levels of government. It also has become a lightning rod for debate over two of the biggest unanswered questions in the American health care debate: Who should receive health care coverage, and who should pay for it?

Those questions take on an added urgency given the emerging interest in using Medicaid as a lever to address social factors, especially housing instability and opioid addiction, that drive poor health outcomes and account for a disproportionate share of health and social service expenditures. This chapter looks more closely at ways in which states and a private insurer are leveraging the Medicaid program to go outside clinic walls and into communities to address those social issues. (Perspectives on the role of Medicaid in providing health care services to immigrant populations appear in Chapter 8, "Achieving Health Equity for Immigrants and Their Children.")

Eliot Fishman lays out the legal framework within which states may use Medicaid funding to promote housing stability among adults and families with multiple barriers to health, including chronic homelessness. Examples from two states illustrate how this works in real-world settings.

James Becker then explains how one state—West Virginia—uses Medicaid to address one of the country's most significant health threats: opioid addiction. Preliminary findings and insights offer a degree of hope while acknowledging the limitations of current strategies.

A Spotlight on myConnections™ illustrates how a major insurer, UnitedHealthcare, concluded that addressing social determinants of health among Medicaid beneficiaries promotes well-being and makes good business sense as well.

Medicaid as a Lever for Social Change

The unique government partnership that drives Medicaid is built on a funding and legal foundation that allows states, Medicaid-funded managed care plans, and providers to go beyond traditional medical care to better manage the health of their beneficiaries. Innovators across the country are developing, testing, and implementing tailored strategies that view health-building activities with a wide lens.

The Funding Framework

Through a shared funding relationship, the federal government reimburses states for most of their Medicaid expenses on a sliding scale, based on a state's per capita income. States with higher per capita incomes receive 50 percent reimbursement, while those with lower per capita incomes are reimbursed at increasingly higher rates. (As of 2019, Mississippi receives the highest federal re-imbursement rate, nearly 78%.)[5] The federal government, however, reimburses states at 90 percent for the services they provide to people in the expanded pool created by the ACA.

Medicaid costs are not spread evenly across enrollees. Setting aside long-term nursing care for frail, elderly, and disabled people, a disproportionate share of Medicaid funds is spent on a relatively small percentage of beneficiaries. Among this vulnerable population are high users of hospital, emergency department, and other costly services. Some cycle in and out of substance misuse or mental illness treatment, experience chronic homelessness, or have complex health problems exacerbated by trauma and poverty. Extending coverage to low-income nondisabled adults thus holds promise for improving health outcomes.

> *The Affordable Care Act brought to Medicaid a population at the intersection of health and human services, prompting greater attention to leveraging Medicaid to address social determinants of health.* —Eliot Fishman

States have financial as well as humane incentives for addressing these challenges. Medicaid accounted for about 28 percent of total state expenditures in federal fiscal year 2015, according to Eliot Fishman, senior director of policy at Families USA. "If you can carve out a few percentage points of savings in Medicaid, you can realize a significant increase in money available for social and other services," he said. Studies have shown, for example, that supportive housing is associated with reduced emergency department use and inpatient hospital admissions, as well as with reduced Medicaid costs.[6]

The Legal Framework

Since its inception, Medicaid has included provisions that allow states to adjust their benefit packages as long as they cover a core set of mandatory services. Beyond those mandates, states can choose from a menu of federally approved optional services and incorporate them into their Medicaid plans.

States can further tailor their programs by requesting federal permission to operate alternative designs or conduct pilot tests. Almost all states, for example, choose to target some services to specific subsets of beneficiaries or structure some or all of their programs around managed care. But states also may deliver additional benefits beyond those listed as statutory options or may otherwise experiment with novel forms of service delivery or payment for services, often by applying for research and demonstration waivers under section 1115 of the Social Security Act.

Both the Medicaid program and the section 1115 waivers were passed at a time of "great ferment and great optimism around social science, the heyday of thinking about community-based solutions to social and economic problems," said Fishman. Because they require evaluations, section 1115 waivers yield an added benefit of identifying and spreading evidence-based practices throughout the country. "The boundaries limiting section 1115 waivers to small pilots have blurred over time, and they are now very much a central part of Medicaid," Fishman added.

Waivers have not traditionally been hotly contested through litigation, but courts are now reviewing some waiver requests that, for example, seek to impose work requirements on beneficiaries or to establish "lockout" periods for individuals who fail to comply with procedural requirements. The fate of this litigation is uncertain, but without a history of judicial precedent on waivers, "we just may have a very different set of legal requirements for Medicaid 1115 waivers by the time this is all done," Fishman observed.

A 2015 bulletin issued by the federal Centers for Medicare and Medicaid Services (CMS) sets out the legal rationale for Medicaid coverage of home and community-based services in general and through waivers.[7]

The CMS bulletin effectively serves as broader guidance for nonmedical services directed at social determinants of health, including not only housing-related services but employment-related services. —Eliot Fishman

Fishman cautioned that informational bulletins are not meant to announce new policy, but rather are intended to summarize and clarify existing policy. States "have to decide how far they can stretch the definitions of 'housing-related activities' and of 'disabilities,' " he explained, and must beware of shifting state-funded services into Medicaid in order to secure federal reimbursement. Recalling his work as an official at CMS, Fishman noted that federal officials view those efforts as inappropriate budget relief, which "creates a real vulnerability for the Medicaid program as a whole."

Fishman highlighted two legal considerations covered by the bulletin, one tied to services and support systems of beneficiaries and the other to payment mechanisms.

Beneficiary Services and Support Systems

Medicaid coverage for home and community-based services has traditionally been tied to the need for institutional care, indicating that a high standard of disability is required. Under the Medicaid statute, these services are limited in some cases to Medicaid beneficiaries leaving nursing homes or more commonly to those living in the community who meet the criteria for a nursing home level of care. Eligibility is therefore determined by individual clinical assessments.

Beneficiaries returning home from an institution might receive support in the form of payment for an apartment security deposit or for essential household furnishings. People already in the community who meet nursing home criteria might receive help in the form of tenancy training or environmental modifications (e.g., wheelchair accommodations) to help them succeed as tenants.

In the past, states have received section 1115 waivers to extend those housing-related services to some at-risk Medicaid beneficiaries, even though they do not meet the high "nursing home level of care" standards of disability, according to Fishman. As larger numbers of at-risk people become eligible for Medicaid under the Affordable Care Act, opportunities open up for states to restructure their systems to address the needs of those beneficiaries in more fundamental ways.

States also have opportunities to request waivers allowing them to use Medicaid funds to pay for planning services. Anticipating that the changed coverage environment would require some significant planning and program adjustments, CMS encouraged a new category of potential Medicaid waivers for state-level coordination and system integration. Establishing these as reimbursable expenses that are not tied to individual clinical assessments opens the door for state experimentation, noted Fishman. Opportunities may exist, for example, to promote state-level data sharing; to break down programmatic and administrative silos between health, housing, and social services systems; and to build the capacity of community-based agencies to work with this population.

Payment Options

Medicaid was established as a fee-for-service payment model and in some locations continues to operate largely that way. Over time, however, most states have chosen to structure all or part of their programs under a system of managed care,[8] many using section 1115 waivers for that authority. Fishman noted two mechanisms available to managed care companies to pay for housing-related activities not otherwise covered as regular Medicaid benefits in that state:

- **"In lieu of" funds:** Managed care plans can sometimes pay for an uncovered service in lieu of a covered one. State approval is required—usually written in the plan's contract—and "in lieu of" services must demonstrate clinical and fiscal benefits. For example, home visits may be covered in lieu of office visits where appropriate.

- **Administrative/margin spending:** After paying for regularly covered medical and "in lieu of" services, managed care companies may purchase goods or services with remaining (margin) funds, based on their judgment that the expense is necessary or that it might prevent a costlier expense. Purchasing an air conditioner for people with asthma is one oft-cited example.

Two States, Two Designs

Several states have cobbled together packages of services using one or more Medicaid waivers to address housing and other nonmedical needs of Medicaid beneficiaries. Fishman highlighted two innovators:

North Carolina

Following a state-initiated overhaul of its Medicaid program in 2015, North Carolina's section 1115 waiver was approved in October 2018, making it one of the first waivers targeted at social determinants of health to be approved under the current administration. The waiver marked the transition of North Carolina's Medicaid program from fee-for-service into managed care, with the goal of integrating physical and behavioral health.

Through the waiver, Medicaid reimbursement became available for enhanced case management and care coordination to improve housing stability, reduce food insecurity, improve access to transportation, and address the consequences of interpersonal violence and toxic stress. These benefits, which had previously been available only to people meeting nursing home care criteria or in some cases to people leaving nursing homes, include:

- *Tenancy services,* such as arranging for a move, paying a security deposit and the first month's rent, assessing the move-in readiness of both the tenant and the unit, and providing help in locating furniture and commodities
- *Housing improvements,* such as remediation for mold or pest infestation
- *Short-term posthospitalization housing* for up to six months
- *Nutrition services* to help secure support from food banks and meal delivery services and to purchase food for specific medical conditions
- *Transportation* that promotes engagement with the community and facilitates participation in services to help people recover from traumatic experiences
- *Child–parent supports* allowing beneficiaries to participate in evidence-based parenting programs

North Carolina is a state to watch, according to Fishman. It has a lot of care co-ordination capacity developed under its fee-for-service system over the past 20 years, and that capacity is migrating into the state's Medicaid managed care system. As of May 2019, North Carolina had not expanded Medicaid eligibility under the Affordable Care Act, a policy that restricts the number of people eligible for the enhanced services.

Massachusetts

Massachusetts, which has a long history with section 1115 waivers, did expand Medicaid under the ACA. The most recent waiver approval, effective November 2016, allows the state to "implement a new Medicaid provider payment structure intended to enable medical providers to engage much more with human services and other community-based organizations," said Fishman.

Under the waiver, beneficiaries of MassHealth (the state's Medicaid program) receive services through newly created Accountable Care Organizations. ACOs are groups of providers that come together voluntarily to offer coordinated, high-quality care to patients that includes a range of health, behavioral, and social services.

ACOs have flexibility in deciding which services they will provide, but reimbursement is tied to performance metrics that get more rigorous over time, as the organizations gain experience under the new system.

> *Massachusetts has thought not only about how the state wants to pay an Accountable Care Organization, but also how it wants individual providers to be paid at the micro-level. —Eliot Fishman*

Examples of services covered under the waiver include:

- *Transition services* for people leaving institutions to live in community settings and community-based services to prevent the need for institutionalization; and *tenancy supports*, such as utility turn-ons or budget training, to promote a safe home environment and sustained tenancy
- *Physical activity and nutrition services* to promote healthy lifestyles
- *Support services for people who have experienced violence*
- *Infrastructure and capacity-building support* to community partner agencies
- *Care management, care coordination, and navigational services*
- *Payments to ACOs* for non-reimbursable services that address health-related social needs
- *Other goods and services* directly related to health and safety

Key issues to watch in Massachusetts, said Fishman, are how broadly the state can define the kinds of services that are available through the Accountable Care Organizations and what sort of clinical assessment, if any, is needed to determine whether a beneficiary is at risk for institutionalization without support services.

Medicaid as a Resource for Reducing Opioid Addiction

States also use section 1115 waivers to test ideas and implement programs related to substance use and mental health. As of June 2019, CMS had approved behavioral health waivers in 28 states, and waivers were pending in 11 more.[9]

Since 2015, when CMS announced guidelines explaining how states can use waivers to expand Medicaid services for people with substance use disorders,[10] they have been embraced by health and human services departments in states that are overwhelmed with the opioid crisis. (This still unfolding tragedy is explored in depth in Chapter 7, "The Opioid Epidemic: Busting Myths and Sharing Solutions.")

Fighting the Opioid Crisis in West Virginia

No state illustrates this pattern or need more clearly than West Virginia, which had the nation's highest drug overdose death rate in 2017 and was one of the first to get a section 1115 waiver to address it. West Virginia is also one of the states that expanded Medicaid eligibility under the ACA.

Officials in the West Virginia Department of Health and Human Resources and its Bureau for Medical Services began working closely with CMS officials on a waiver request aimed at combating substance use among newly Medicaid-eligible West Virginia residents.[11] The goals were to increase the availability of substance use disorder prevention and treatment services and to create a continuum of care.

Once the waiver was approved in October 2017, West Virginia expanded services for Medicaid recipients in two phases to include:[12]

- **Screening, Brief Intervention, and Referral to Treatment (SBIRT)**: West Virginia implemented statewide use of this widely accepted tool to identify needs among individuals in the Medicaid population with substance use challenges.
- **Methadone treatment and administration:** The state added Medicaid coverage for methadone as a withdrawal management strategy, for administering

and monitoring the medication, and for all-important counseling-related services.

- **Naloxone distribution:** The state designed and implemented a statewide initiative to make naloxone widely available to Medicaid beneficiaries; reimburse providers for using naloxone in their treatment programs; and increase awareness of the benefits of the drug, which can reverse the effects of an opioid overdose if administered in a timely manner.
- **Reimbursement for all levels of short-term residential treatment, peer recovery support services, and withdrawal management:** These services include enhanced targeted case management services as Medicaid beneficiaries move from institutional settings back into the community, as well as intensive outpatient care.

What the West Virginia Data Show

Although early data is limited (phase 1 of the initiative began in January 2018; phase 2 began in July 2018), Becker has identified some trends in the treatment of substance use disorders.

One of the most important things about the waiver, he said, is that it allows Medicaid to pay for methadone programs, which has helped to establish the drug as part of a medical model of care, rather than as something separate and often somewhat hidden.

"In the past, it was just something nobody spoke about. The patients just went to the clinics, they got their methadone, and their doctor probably didn't even know they got it unless they actually did a drug test," said Becker. That has changed with the availability of Medicaid coverage, which also "allows us to look at comparative data between methadone, buprenorphine, and naltrexone [three FDA-approved medications to manage opioid dependence] to determine whether one or the other is better treatment."

Methadone programs in West Virginia treat some 8,000 individuals statewide, with about 1,800 of those individuals covered by Medicaid. In many cases, these programs have stabilized these at-risk patients for a long time. "I have had three patients who have been involved with the methadone treatment program since they returned from Vietnam," said Becker.

He cautioned, however, that there are too few medication-assisted treatment providers participating in Medicaid to meet the need in West Virginia. While approximately 700 providers are certified to provide buprenorphine treatment in the state, Becker noted that only about half of them currently accept Medicaid. A significant number continue to operate in "cash-only" settings, which Becker believes poses numerous problems. "Personally, I think we shouldn't view the care of this unfortunate population as a chance to get rich," he commented frankly.

Despite the challenges, having Medicaid-approved providers allows state and local health departments to collect data. When that information is available, said Becker, "I can tell you what their average daily dose is. I can tell you when they've brought their average daily dose down, and that they're getting counseling. So that's a big step under our waiver."

> It's so important to get good data from all the sources of treatment.
> —James Becker

Becker is less certain about the benefits of other waiver services, including adding 600 residential beds to the 200 that are currently available. "The benefit of those residential services is really unclear to me, because data to support the effectiveness is lacking," he acknowledged. He suggested that a short-term stay for detoxification, closely coupled with referrals to outpatient services, might be more valuable.

He also expressed reservations about SBIRT, acknowledging that he had not seen the hoped-for benefits. "While I have respect for those endorsing SBIRT, I have concerns that the treatment component has achieved less than we desire. While SBIRT has clearly been a benefit in treating alcohol use, it has been more challenging in opioid use disorder. If these patients have to wait more than 48 hours, they frequently lose their focus and they don't get to treatment."

Becker is more confident of the value of peer recovery support services, where an overdose report triggers an assessment from a quick response team. Within 24 hours, someone from peer recovery support services has made direct contact with the individual who overdosed and is working to connect that person to treatment. "That has really helped increase the number of people getting into treatment services," Becker said. Since using the quick response team approach, Becker reports a 33 percent reduction in overdoses in his area of practice.

RWJF has recognized the value of peer support for opioid users as well. The Foundation sponsored an Opioid Challenge to help create technology to support and connect individuals affected by opioid addiction. The 2018 Opioid Challenge winner was Sober Grid, a mobile app platform that connects substance users with a community of peers for support and includes features to help users manage their addiction.[13]

The expanded availability of naloxone to families of prescription opioid users and to all first responders also has had clear benefits. "The data shows that giving naloxone in the field clearly reduces the number of people who get intubated in the ER, and it saves some lives," Becker confirmed. "This means they are not going to be as critically ill when they get to the ER and some can be treated there and discharged with follow-up without being admitted."

Although many other states are considering the benefits of section 1115 waivers to help diminish the opioid crisis, Becker is far from certain that West Virginia has turned the corner on the problem. "I'm still a long way from having a lot of hope but I do believe that we are bending the curve," he said. "We're beginning to understand the scope of the problem differently. I think the waiver is definitely a significant part of that."

A Final Word

Medicaid affords Americans of all ages opportunities to be healthy and live independently. It promotes health equity by helping children grow and thrive, enabling disabled people to remain in their homes as long as they can, and offering long-term nursing care when living at home is no longer possible. It is not surprising, then, that Medicaid emerged as a priority within RWJF's Transforming Health and Health Care Systems area of focus, which, according to the Foundation, "will have a principal, but not exclusive, focus on people eligible for Medicaid."

RWJF's attention to this area is essential because the opportunities available through the size and flexibility of Medicaid have always rendered it a complex and controversial program, filled with arcane language and riddled with service and coverage gaps, especially given the profound challenges of many beneficiaries.

System reforms available through waivers and the Affordable Care Act have allowed states to start filling some of those gaps. Waivers stem from an American tradition that values decentralized control and "cooperative federalism," and the Affordable Care Act and subsequent waiver approvals build on an emerging awareness that social and economic circumstances drive health as much as, or more than, clinical care.

Now that 75 percent of the states have opted to take advantage of the Medicare expansion, Fishman hopes the question of access to coverage is moving closer to resolution. But a tangle of questions remain about how best to juggle the multiple pressures and opportunities still at hand. "Providing Medicaid coverage is a necessary but not sufficient condition that triggers all of the other reforms we have been talking about," he said.

The significant infrastructure and start-up costs involved in implementing Medicaid reforms loom as potential barriers. Health care and social service providers will need to develop new information systems, recruit and retrain providers, and establish data-exchange protocols in order to realize the benefits from the federal infusion of new money into Medicaid. Absent resources to cover those expenses, some states are unlikely to have the capacity to make the sweeping improvements envisioned by waivers or other mechanisms.

Identifying and implementing the most promising policies, targeting funds where they will be most effective, ensuring that resources are adequate to achieve the goals, and accomplishing all of that within budgetary and political constraints remain the challenges of the future.

Chapter 11 Spotlight: A Private Insurer Tackles Social Determinants

Ana Fuentevilla, MD, MHCDS, Chief Medical Officer, Optum Population Health Solutions (former Chief Medical Officer, UnitedHealthcare Community & State).

UnitedHealthcare (UHC) provides health coverage to nearly 49 million people in the United States and around the world,[1] including 6.7 million Medicaid beneficiaries who live in 30 states and Washington, DC. Medicaid members receive coverage through a system of managed care overseen by the company's Community & State division.

Health Care Does Not Guarantee Good Health

Although it offers state-of-the-art clinical and other health services, UHC was not satisfied with the health outcomes of some of its most vulnerable members. Too many were cycling in and out of hospitals and emergency departments, presenting with a complex array of health challenges. Yet their high use of care was not making them healthy.

> *We would be doing our jobs well if we can help our Medicaid members get back on their feet, find a purpose. We think of that as a Culture of Health and as success. —Ana Fuentevilla[2]*

Prior UHC efforts offered some guidance in helping its vulnerable members fare better. The company had a history of providing its elderly Medicare members with supports that allowed them to remain in their homes, and staff saw that those supports made a measurable difference. UHC believed that addressing housing and other nonclinical needs had the potential to yield good outcomes for its nonelderly beneficiaries as well.

The company began to dive more deeply into the complex needs and outcomes of its Medicaid beneficiaries, starting by identifying the constellation of social determinants that posed the most serious obstacles to their well-being. Clinical data "hot-spotting"—UHC's systematic analysis of members' health records, patterns of health care utilization, and health care costs—provided a partial answer. Publicly available community and demographic data added detail and nuance.

Three problems—housing, transportation, and employment—stood out, with housing emerging as the most consequential in terms of its impact on the overall health of members, their use of health care services, and the opportunity for better long-term outcomes. For example, Medicaid members experiencing homelessness in Maricopa County, the setting for the 2018 Sharing Knowledge conference, used the emergency room nine times more often, were hospitalized six times more frequently, and incurred three times more health care expenses than other Medicaid members living in Arizona.

Addressing the root causes of homelessness sparked a new venture for UHC— myConnections™—which was launched in select communities throughout the country in 2016.

myConnections

There are three core commitments to myConnections: the program is designed to be community-based and data-driven, and to provide a housing and social service solution for low-income members who were frequent users of the health care system. Focused initially on members experiencing homelessness or housing insecurity, the program expanded in 2017 to serve members coming out of prison, pregnant women and new mothers struggling with addiction, and those who are frail and homebound.

myConnections in Action

A key contributor to the success of myConnections has been UHC's strategic partnership with Chicanos Por La Causa, a Phoenix-based social services and community development agency. The two organizations share a goal of helping individuals and families with low or moderate income secure and retain quality, affordable housing. Through the partnership UHC committed to providing Chicanos Por La Causa access to up to $20 million of capital to acquire, develop, and operate multifamily housing units in the Phoenix area, as well as to oversee a variety of need-based services to residents.

Amy's Story

For years Amy, age 26, turned to drugs and alcohol to numb the emotional effects of multiple family tragedies. Her lowest point, she says, was when she was arrested for possession while living on the streets, and she learned in jail that she was pregnant. Amy knew she had to make a life change and was able to enroll in a treatment program for homeless pregnant and parenting women at an organization that partners with myConnections.

Today, Amy lives with her baby girl in a set-aside apartment in an affordable housing community—a safe and stable place where she can love and nurture her baby while she works on healing herself. She has the integrated support and encouragement of a health coach, behavioral health therapist, and employment navigator as she completes probation and outpatient treatment, and then plans her transition to living independently, in permanent housing, as a contributing member of society.

Now 20 months sober, Amy beams with pride about how far she's come. She's earning an income at a new job and is looking forward to attending community college this fall. She prays and meditates to stay focused on her sobriety and on being the best mom possible.

Achieving the Triple Aim

UHC is acting on the recognition that when social determinants of health are proactively addressed, members' health improves, and total cost of care is often reduced. By investing in myConnections, UHC is participating in a societal effort to transform traditional clinical care into a tool that focuses on the whole person and achieves the triple aim—better care, better health, lower costs.

The story of another UHC member highlights what is possible. Tom had visited the emergency department more than 200 times in the year after losing his home, accruing health care expenditures of nearly $200,000. After living in stable set-aside housing, supported by counseling and other social services through myConnections, Tom's health-care utilization dropped dramatically, allowing him to focus on goals and gradually gain the confidence he needed to sustain his journey back to better health and well-being.

Given its long-term commitment to the communities it serves, UHC no longer considers myConnections a pilot program. As of February 2019, Arizona, Hawaii, Michigan, Nebraska, Nevada, and Wisconsin were operating myConnections programs, and more states are in the pipeline.

Conclusion

"Whatever affects one directly affects all indirectly," wrote Martin Luther King Jr. in his "Letter from a Birmingham Jail," and that insight remains resonant as RWJF advances toward a Culture of Health. Without discounting the depth of the challenges that could slow that journey, both the *Sharing Knowledge* conference and this book build on the conviction that "we, not me" is the best way forward.

A year after this conference, RWJF convened another intersectional meeting, this time in Houston, Tex. It was impossible not to reflect on the changes that had occurred in the interim, as immigration grew into a heated controversy in those two border states and beyond.

At least in part, one narrative had become dominant over others, which is why RWJF is reflecting more on which stories get told, how they alter mind-sets, and what actions result. We have renewed our resolve to highlight connections, rather than differences, when we talk about common problems, and to take evidence-based action grounded in that shared understanding.

Despite an abundance of political rhetoric, there is ample enthusiasm for doing just that, as this book has shown. A cross-sectional movement to address climate change is on the rise, bringing together businesses, hospitals, and activists. The opioid epidemic and its intersections with rural health and mass incarceration are gaining attention across partisan divides. Medical systems are integrating the social determinants of health into their care interventions, and novel payer initiatives are making it feasible to pilot test and evaluate innovation. Resilience also has come to the forefront as we learn more about the risks associated with childhood trauma, weather-related and human-spawned disasters, and community fragmentation, as well as the protective factors that can counter those stressors and foster personal and collective renewal.

The pursuit of health equity remains the underpinning of everything we do. As RWJF explores further the cultural aspect of a Culture of Health, we are

Culture of Health in Practice, Alonzo L. Plough. Oxford University Press (2020) © Robert Wood Johnson Foundation
DOI: 10.1093/oso/9780190071400.001.0001

bolstering our commitment to empower historically marginalized people. The data, stories, and analyses in this book give voice to those who have been most affected by inequities as they chart broadly inclusive pathways toward health. Look for future volumes in the Culture of Health series to track the continued evolution of RWJF's work, and the power of cross-cutting partnerships to provide everyone that fair and just opportunity to be healthier.

ACKNOWLEDGMENTS

The *Sharing Knowledge to Build a Culture of Health* conference involved the hard work of numerous individuals, both internal and external to the Robert Wood Johnson Foundation (RWJF). Priya Gandhi led the successful development of the conference in collaboration with Lisa Simpson and her staff at AcademyHealth. I also would like to thank the external steering committee who helped develop the conference sessions.

Turning the third annual conference into this volume also required the vision and support of many. An Editorial Review Group oversees the development of this series and provided careful commentary and suggestions. My colleagues in this group are Sandro Galea, Boston University; Sherry Glied, New York University; Frederick Mann, Robert Wood Johnson Foundation; and Chad Zimmerman, Oxford University Press.

Additional thanks to the team at RWJF who provided essential leadership throughout the development of this manuscript: Priya Gandhi, Ed Ghisu, Sofia Kounelias, Brian Quinn, and Kristin Silvani.

Finally, with guidance from RWJF staff, a team of talented writers crafted the manuscript, weaving together multiple data sources, including conference presentations and interviews, into cross-cutting chapters that reflect the conference objectives. Thank you to Karyn Feiden, Mary B. Geisz, Margaret O. Kirk, and Mary Nakashian.

REFERENCES

Introduction

1. Braverman P, Arkin E, Orleans T, et al., "What Is Health Equity? And What Difference Does a Definition Make?" Robert Wood Johnson Foundation, May 1, 2017, https://www.rwjf.org/en/library/research/2017/05/what-is-health-equity-.html.
2. Murphy SL, Xu JQ, Kochanek KD, et al., "Mortality in the United States, 2017," NCHS Data Brief no. 328, National Center for Health Statistics, 2018, https://www.cdc.gov/nchs/products/databriefs/db328.htm.

Section I

1. Gandhi M, *India of My Dreams* (Ahmedabad: Jitendra T. Desai and Navajivan Mudranalaya, 1947), https://www.mkgandhi.org/ebks/India-Dreams.pdf.

Chapter 1

1. Frey WH, "The US Will Become 'Minority White' in 2045, Census Projects," Brookings, The Avenue, *www.brookings.edu/blog/the-avenue/2018/03/14/the-us-will-become-minority-white-in-2045-census-projects/*.
2. "Fast Facts," IES/NCES, National Center for Education Statistics, *www.nces.ed.gov/fastfacts/*.
3. Bialik K, "For the Fifth Time in a Row, the New Congress Is the Most Racially and Ethnically Diverse Ever," Pew Research Center, Fact Tank, February 8, 2019, *www.pewresearch.org/fact-tank/2019/02/08/for-the-fifth-time-in-a-row-the-new-congress-is-the-most-racially-and-ethnically-diverse-ever/*.
4. "Quick Facts: Arizona," U.S. Census Bureau, *www.census.gov/quickfacts/az*.
5. Ruiz JM, Sbarra D, and Steffen PR, "Hispanic Ethnicity, Stress Psychophysiology, and Paradoxical Health Outcomes: A Review with Conceptual Considerations and a Call for Research," *International Journal of Psychophysiology* 131 (September 2018): 24–29, abstract at *www.sciencedirect.com/science/article/abs/pii/S0167876017304786*.
6. "Hispanic Heritage Month 2018," U.S. Census Bureau, Newsroom, release no. CB18-FF.07, *www.census.gov/newsroom/facts-for-features/2018/hispanic-heritage-month.html*.
7. "Facts on U.S. Latinos 2015," Pew Research Center, September 18, 2017, *www.pewhispanic.org/2017/09/18/facts-on-u-s-latinos/*.
8. "Profile: Hispanic/Latino Americans," U.S. Department of Health and Human Services, Office of Minority Health, *https://minorityhealth.hhs.gov/omh/browse.aspx?lvl=3&lvlid=64*.
9. Ibid.

10. "Health, United States 2016," U.S. Department of Health and Human Services, Centers for Disease Control and Prevention, National Center for Health Statistics, *www.cdc.gov/nchs/data/hus/hus16.pdf*.

11. "National Vital Statistics Reports: United States Life Tables, 2015," Centers for Disease Control and Prevention, vol. 67, no. 7, November 13, 2018, *www.cdc.gov/nchs/data/nvsr/nvsr67/nvsr67_07-508.pdf*.

12. Ruiz JM, Hamann HA, Mehl MR, et al., "The Hispanic Health Paradox: From Epidemiological Phenomenon to Contribution Opportunities for Psychological Science," *Group Processes & Intergroup Relations*, April 2016, abstract at *https://journals.sagepub.com/doi/abs/10.1177/1368430216638540?journalCode=gpia*.

13. "Infant Mortality Rates by Race and Ethnicity, 2016," Centers for Disease Control and Prevention, *www.cdc.gov/reproductivehealth/maternalinfanthealth/infantmortality.htm#chart*.

14. "Infant Mortality and Hispanic Americans," Centers for Disease Control and Prevention, Office of Minority Health, *https://minorityhealth.hhs.gov/omh/browse.aspx?lvl=4&lvlid=68*.

15. "Profile: Hispanic/Latino Americans," U.S. Department of Health and Human Services, Office of Minority Health, *https://minorityhealth.hhs.gov/omh/browse.aspx?lvl=3&lvlid=64*

16. Ruiz JM, Campos B, and Garcia JJ, "Introduction to the Special Issue on Latino Physical Health: Disparities, Paradoxes, and Future Directions," *Journal of Latino Psychology* 4, no. 2 (2016): 61–66, *https://psycnet.apa.org/fulltext/2016-21991-001.html*.

17. Arias E, Eschbach K, Schauman WS, et al., "The Hispanic Mortality Advantage and Ethnic Misclassification on U.S. Death Certificates," *American Journal of Public Health* 100, no. S1 (April 1, 2010): S171–S177, *https://doi.org/10.2105/AJPH.2008.135863*.

18. Ruiz JM, Steffen P, and Smith TB, "Hispanic Mortality Paradox: A Systematic Review and Analysis of the Longitudinal Literature," *American Journal of Public Health* 103, no. 3 (January 2017): e52–60, abstract at *www.ncbi.nlm.nih.gov/pubmed/23327278*.

19. The American Community Survey is an ongoing survey of the Census Bureau, providing annual information about jobs, education, veteran status, housing, and other topics, *www.census.gov/programs-surveys/acs/about.html*.

20. Holt-Lunstad J, Smith TB, and Layton JB, "Social Relationships and Mortality Risk: A Meta-Analytic Review," *PLoS Med* 7, no. 7 (July 27, 2010): e1000316, *www.ncbi.nlm.nih.gov/pmc/articles/PMC2910600/*.

21. These terms, or variations of them, appear in several studies. Calzada EJ, Fernandez Y, and Cortes DE, for example, published a study of *respeto*, "Incorporating the Cultural Value of Respeto Into a Framework of Latino Parenting," *Cultural Diversity & Ethnic Minority Psychology* 16, no. 1 (January 2010): 77–86, *www.ncbi.nlm.nih.gov/pmc/articles/PMC4403003/*.

    The value of *familismo* appears in Campos B, Schetter CD, Abdou CM, et al., "Familialism, Social Support, and Stress: Positive Implications for Pregnant Latinas," *Cultural Diversity & Ethnic Minority Psychology* 14, no. 2 (April 2008): 155–62, abstract at *https://psycnet.apa.org/doiLanding?doi=10.1037%2F1099-9809.14.2.155*.

    Simpatica and *familismo* appear in Ma M, Malcolm LR, Diaz-Albertini K, et al., "Cultural Assets and Substance Use Among Hispanic Adolescents," *Health Education Behavior* 44, no. 2 (April 2017): 326–31, abstract at *www.ncbi.nlm.nih.gov/pubmed/27450551*.

22. Shar RJ and Pickett KE, "The Health Benefits of Hispanic Communities for Non-Hispanic Mothers and Infants: Another Hispanic Paradox," *American Journal of Public Health*, published online May 9, 2013, abstract at *https://ajph.aphapublications.org/doi/10.2105/AJPH.2012.300985*.

23. Coan JA and Sbarra DA, "Social Baseline Theory: The Social Regulation of Risk and Effort," *Current Opinion in Psychology* 1 (February 2015): 87–91, abstract at *www.sciencedirect.com/science/article/pii/S2352250X14000396*.

24. Campos, et al., "Familialism."

25. "The Need: A Civilization Disrupted," Native Americans in Philanthropy, *https://nativephilanthropy.org/the-need/*.

26. Ibid.

27. "American Fact Finder," U.S. Census Bureau, *https://factfinder.census.gov/faces/tableservices/jsf/pages/productview.xhtml?src=bkmk*.

28. "Frequently Asked Questions," U.S. Department of the Interior, Bureau of Indian Affairs, *www.bia.gov/frequently-asked-questions*.
29. "Profile: American Indian/Alaska Native," U.S. Department of Health and Human Services, Office of Minority Affairs, *https://minorityhealth.hhs.gov/omh/browse.aspx?lvl=3&lvlid=62*.
30. Gonzalez R, Yellow Bird M, and Walters K, "The Indigenous Lifecourse: Strengthening the Health and Well-Being of Native Youth," Native Americans in Philanthropy, 2016, *www.nativephilanthropy.org/wp-content/uploads/2015/11/Indigenous-Lifecourse-NAP-Report.pdf*.
31. LEED certification, administered by the U.S. Green Building Council, is a globally recognized rating system for sustainability.

Chapter 2

1. Pribble JM, Goldstein KM, Fowler EF, et al. "Medical News for the Public to Use: What's on Local TV News?" *American Journal of Managed Care* 12, no. 3 (March 2006): 170–76.
2. Gollust SE, Fowler EF, and Niederdeppe J, "Television News Coverage of Public Health Issues and Implications for Public Health Policy and Practice," *Annual Review of Public Health* 40 (April 2019): 167–85.
3. Gollust SE and Lantz PM, "Communicating Population Health: Print News Media Coverage of Type 2 Diabetes," *Social Science & Medicine* 69, no. 7 (October 2009): 1091–98, doi: 10.1016/j.socscimed.2009.07.009.
4. Nagler RH, Bigman CA, Ramanadhan S, et al., "Prevalence and Framing of Health Disparities in Local Print News: Implications for Multilevel Interventions to Address Cancer Inequalities," *Cancer Epidemiology, Biomarkers, & Prevention* 25, no. 4 (April 2016): 603–12. www.ncbi.nlm.nih.gov/pubmed/27196094
5. Fowler EF, Baum LM, Barry C, et al., "Media Messages and Perceptions of the Affordable Care Act During the Early Phase of Implementation," *Journal of Health Politics, Policy and Law* 42, no. 1 (2017): 167–95.
6. Ibid.
7. Karaca-Mandic P, Wilcock A, Baum L, et al., "The Volume of TV Advertisements During the ACA's First Enrollment Period Was Associated With Increased Insurance Coverage," *Health Affairs* 36, no. 4 (April 2017): https://doi.org/10.1377/hlthaff.2016.1440.
8. Niederdeppe J, Fowler EF, Goldstein K, et al., "Does Local Television News Coverage Cultivate Fatalistic Beliefs About Cancer Prevention?" *Journal of Communication* 60 (2010): 230–53.
9. Niederdeppe J, Lee T, Robbins R, et al., "Content and Effects of News Stories About Uncertain Cancer Causes and Preventive Behaviors," *Health Communication* 29 (2014): 332–46.
10. Kennedy-Hendricks A, Barry CL, and Gollust SE, "Social Stigma Toward Persons With Prescription Opioid Use Disorder: Associations With Public Support for Punitive and Public Health–Oriented Policies," *Psychiatric Services* 68, no. 5 (2017): 462–69.
11. Gollust SE, Barry CL, and Niederdeppe J, "Partisan Responses to Public Health Messages: Motivated Reasoning and Sugary Drink Taxes," *Journal of Health Politics, Policy and Law* 42, no. 6 (2017): 1005–37.
12. Harris JL, Frazier W, Romo-Palafox M, et al., "F.A.C.T.S. 2017: Food Industry Regulation After 10 Years: Progress and Opportunities to Improve Food Advertising to Children," UConn Rudd Center for Food Policy & Obesity, November 2017, http://www.uconnruddcenter.org/files/Pdfs/FACTS-2017_Final.pdf.
13. Centers for Disease Control and Prevention, National Center for Chronic Disease Prevention and Health Promotion (NCCDPHP), "Our Budget," https://www.cdc.gov/chronicdisease/programs-impact/budget/index.htm.
14. Gollust SE, Fowler EF, and Niederdeppe J, "Television News Coverage of Public Health Issues and Implications for Public Health Policy and Practice."
15. Gollust SE, Bauma LM, Niederdeppe J, et al., "Local Television News Coverage of the Affordable Care Act: Emphasizing Politics Over Consumer Information," *American Journal of Public Health* (May 1, 2017): https://ajph.aphapublications.org/doi/10.2105/AJPH.2017.303659.

16. Shearer E, "Social Media Outpaces Print Newspapers in the U.S. as a News Source," Pew Research Center, Fact Tank, December 10, 2018, http://www.pewresearch.org/fact-tank/2018/12/10/social-media-outpaces-print-newspapers-in-the-u-s-as-a-news-source.
17. Gyenes N and Mina AX, "How Misinfodemics Spread Disease," *The Atlantic*, August 30, 2018, https://www.theatlantic.com/technology/archive/2018/08/how-misinfodemics-spread-disease/568921/.
18. Weeks BE, "Media and Political Misperceptions," in *Misinformation and Mass Audiences*, ed. Southwell BG, Thorson EA, and Sheble L. Austin: University of Texas Press, 2018, page 141.
19. Seymour B, Gyenes N, Robert H, et al., "Public Health, Social Networks, and the Digital Media Ecosystem: Emerging Hypotheses," Substance Abuse Library and Information Studies, *Proceedings of the 39th Annual SALIS/AMHL Conference*, Worcester, MA, 2017, 5–9.
20. Gollust SE, Bauma LM, Niederdeppe J, et al., "Local Television News Coverage of the Affordable Care Act: Emphasizing Politics Over Consumer Information," *American Journal of Public Health* (May 1, 2017): https://ajph.aphapublications.org/doi/10.2105/AJPH.2017.303659.
21. Gyenes N, PowerPoint presentation prepared for RWJF's Sharing Knowledge conference, Phoenix, Arizona, March 2018.
22. Vosoughi S, Roy D, and Aral S, "The Spread of True and False News Online," *Science*, March 9, 2018. https://science.sciencemag.org/content/359/6380/1146.

Chapter 2 Spotlight: Media Marketing to Minority Youth

1. Harris JL, Shehan C, Gross R, et al., "Food Advertising Targeted to Hispanic and Black Youth: Contributing to Health Disparities," Rudd Report, 2015, http://www.uconnruddcenter.org/files/Pdfs/272-7%20%20Rudd_Targeted%20Marketing%20Report_Release_081115%5B1%5D.pdf.
2. Ibid.
3. Harris JL, Frazier W, Kumanyika S, et al., "Increasing Disparities in Unhealthy Food Advertising Targeted to Hispanic and Black Youth," Rudd Report, 2019, http://uconnruddcenter.org/files/Pdfs/TargetedMarketingReport2019.pdf.
4. Hyary M and Harris JL, "Hispanic Youth Visits to Food and Beverage Company Websites," *Health Equity* 1, no. 1 (2018): 134–38.
5. Fleming-Milici F and Harris JL, "Liking, Sharing, and Following: Adolescents' Engagement With Unhealthy Food and Beverage Brands on Social Media," unpublished manuscript, 2019.
6. Harris JL, Frazier W, Fleming-Milici F, et al., "A Qualitative Assessment of Black and Latino Adolescents' Attitudes About Targeted Marketing of Unhealthy Food and Beverages," unpublished manuscript, 2019.

Section II

1. The Robert Wood Johnson Foundation has dedicated significant resources to the important role of play in achieving a Culture of Health, through such programs as Active Living by Design and Playworks. For more information, see https://www.rwjf.org/en/library/research/2011/10/active-living-by-design.html and https://www.rwjf.org/en/library/research/2017/09/the-scaling-of-playworks--a-case-study.html.

Chapter 3

1. Badger K, "In Rural America, Community-Driven Solutions Improve Health," Robert Wood Johnson Foundation, Blog, November 15, 2017, https://www.rwjf.org/en/blog/2017/11/rural-america-healthier-with-community-driven-solutions.html.
2. "Life in Rural America," National Public Radio, the Robert Wood Johnson Foundation, the Harvard T. H. Chan School of Public Health, October 1, 2018, https://www.rwjf.org/content/dam/farm/reports/surveys_and_polls/2018/rwjf449263.

3. "Rural Health and Well-Being in America," Robert Wood Johnson Foundation, https://www.rwjf.org/en/library/collections/rural-health-in-america. html?rid=003E000001Pe9sKIAR&et_cid=1532461.
4. Porter E, "The Hard Truths of Trying to 'Save' the Rural Economy," *New York Times*, December 14, 2018, https://www.nytimes.com/interactive/2018/12/14/opinion/rural-america-trump-decline.html?rref=collection%2Fbyline%2Feduardo-porter&auth=login-email&module=inline.
5. Coe WK, "The Rural Heartbeat," *Daily Yonder*, December 19, 2018, http://www.dailypostathenian.com/opinion/article_a3e043a6-627c-5347-b8d3-7f4cc69c8ef5.html.
6. U.S. Census Bureau, 1910 to 1990 Censuses, www.census.gov/population/censusdata/urpop0090.txt; 2000 decennial census, Table P002; 2010 decennial census, Table P2.
7. "What Works? Strategies to Improve Rural Health," County Health Rankings & Roadmaps, Robert Wood Johnson Foundation, http://www.countyhealthrankings.org/what-works-strategies-improve-rural-health.
8. "Life in Rural America."
9. Porter, "Hard Truths of Trying to 'Save' the Rural Economy."
10. "What Works?"
11. "Why Education Matters to Health: Exploring the Causes," VCU Center on Society and Health and the Robert Wood Johnson Foundation, April 2014, https://www.rwjf.org/content/dam/farm/reports/issue_briefs/2014/rwjf412692.
12. U.S. Census Bureau, "Percentage of People in Poverty," https://www2.census.gov/programs-surveys/demo/tables/p60/263/statepov.xls.
13. Tye L, Bobby Kennedy: The Making of a Liberal Icon (New York: Random House, 2016), 349.
14. "About Us," HOPE (Hope Enterprise Corporation and Hope Credit Union), https://hopecu.org/about/.
15. "The Tapestry of Black Business Ownership in America: Untapped Opportunities for Success," Association for Enterprise Opportunity, February 16, 2017, https://www.aeoworks.org/wp-content/uploads/2019/03/AEO_Black_Owned_Business_Report_02_16_17_FOR_WEB.pdf.
16. Schlegel R and Peng S, "As the South Grows: On Fertile Soil," National Committee for Responsive Philanthropy, April 4, 2017, https://www.ncrp.org/publication/as-the-south-grows-on-fertile-soil.
17. "Mission," Center for Rural Strategies, https://www.ruralstrategies.org/mission-1/.
18. "Strengthening and Coordinating Local Leadership Networks Across Rural Places to Address Long-Standing Inequity and Historic Trauma," Center for Rural Strategies, Robert Wood Johnson Foundation Grant ID no. 75992.
19. Houk R, "Connecting Rural Tennessee to Broadband," *Johnson City Press*, September 19, 2018, https://www.johnsoncitypress.com/Business/2018/09/19/Connecting-rural-Tennessee-to-broadband.
20. Jordan M, "ICE Came for a Tennessee Town's Immigrants. The Town Fought Back," *New York Times*, June 8, 2018, https://www.nytimes.com/interactive/2018/06/11/us/tennessee-immigration-trump.html
21. "Poll: Four in Ten Rural Americans Report Problems Paying for Medical Bills, Housing, or Food; Majority Optimistic About Having an Impact on Improving Their Communities," Robert Wood Johnson Foundation, May 21, 2019, https://www.rwjf.org/en/library/articles-and-news/2019/05/four-in-ten-rural-americans-report-problems-paying-for-medical-bills-housing-or-food.html.

Chapter 4

1. Michael S, Merlo C, Basch C, et al., "Critical Connections: Health and Academics," *Journal of School Health* 85, no. 11 (2015): 740–58, https://www.ncbi.nlm.nih.gov/pmc/articles/PMC4606776/.
2. U.S. Census Bureau, 2013–2017 American Community Survey, https://www.census.gov/programs-surveys/acs/technical-documentation/table-and-geography-changes/2017/5-year.html.

3. Highlights from *The Condition of Education 2017* (Washington, DC: National Center for Education Statistics, 2018), https://nces.ed.gov/programs/coe/indicator_coi.asp.

4. *National Assessment of Educational Progress—The Nation's Report Card: Mathematics & Reading at Grade 12* (Washington, DC: National Center for Education Statistics, 2015), https://www.nationsreportcard.gov/reading_math_g12_2015/#.

5. Ibid.

6. U.S. Census Bureau, "2016 American Community Survey 1-Year Estimates, Poverty Status in the Past 12 Months," 2017, https://factfinder.census.gov.

7. U.S. Census Bureau, 2018 Current Population Survey, 2018, https://www.census.gov/data/tables/2018/demo/families/cps-2018.html.

8. USDA Economic Research Service, "2017 Current Population Survey Food Security Supplement," 2017, https://www.ers.usda.gov/topics/food-nutrition-assistance/food-security-in-the-us/key-statistics-graphics.aspx.

9. Cree RA, Bitsko RH, Robinson LR, et al., "Health Care, Family, and Community Factors Associated With Mental, Behavioral, and Developmental Disorders and Poverty Among Children Aged 2–8 Years—United States, 2016," *MMWR Weekly Report* 67, no. 5 (2018): 1377–83, https://www.cdc.gov/mmwr/volumes/67/wr/mm6750a1.htm.

10. Ghandour RM, Sherman LJ, Vladutiu CJ, et al., "Prevalence and Treatment of Depression, Anxiety, and Conduct Problems in U.S. Children," *Journal of Pediatrics* 206 (2019): 256–67, https://www.ncbi.nlm.nih.gov/pubmed/30322701.

11. Perou R, Bitsko RH, Blumberg SJ, et al., "Mental Health Surveillance Among Children: United States, 2005–2011," *MMWR* 62(Supplement) (2013): 1–35, https://www.cdc.gov/mmwr/preview/mmwrhtml/su6202a1.htm.

12. Kann LK, McManus T, Harris WA, et al., "Youth Risk Behavior Surveillance—United States 2017," *MMWR Surveillance Summaries* 67, no. 8 (2018): 1–114, https://www.cdc.gov/mmwr/volumes/67/ss/ss6708a1.htm.

13. U.S. Administration for Children & Families, "Child Maltreatment 2017," 2019, https://www.acf.hhs.gov/cb/resource/child-maltreatment-2017.

14. Ibid.

15. Metzler M, Merrick MT, Klevens J, et al., "Adverse Childhood Experiences and Life Opportunities: Shifting the Narrative," *Children and Youth Services Review* 72 (2017): 141–49, https://www.sciencedirect.com/science/article/pii/S0190740916303449.

16. Sacks V and Murphey D, "The Prevalence of Adverse Childhood Experiences, Nationally, by State, and by Race or Ethnicity," Child Trends, February 20, 2018, https://www.childtrends.org/publications/prevalence-adverse-childhood-experiences-nationally-state-race-ethnicity.

17. National Center for Chronic Disease Prevention and Health Promotion, Centers for Disease Control and Prevention, "Health and Academic Achievement," May 2014, https://www.cdc.gov/healthyschools/health_and_academics/pdf/health-academic-achievement.pdf.

18. Michael, Merlo, Basch, et al., "Critical Connections: Health and Academics."

19. Rasberry CN, Tiu, GF, Kann L, et al., "Health-Related Behaviors and Academic Achievement Among High School Students—United States, 2015," *MMWR Weekly Report* 66, no. 35 (2017): 921–27, https://www.cdc.gov/mmwr/volumes/66/wr/mm6635a1.htm.

20. Kann, McManus, and Harris, "Youth Risk Behavior Surveillance."

21. Lohrmann DK, "A Complementary Ecological Model of the Coordinated School Health Program," *Public Health Reports* 123, no. 6 (2008): 695–703, https://www.ncbi.nlm.nih.gov/pmc/articles/PMC2556714/.

22. ASCD, *The Learning Compact Redefined: A Call to Action* (Alexandria, VA: ASCD, 2007), http://www.ascd.org/ASCD/pdf/Whole%20Child/WCC%20Learning%20Compact.pdf.

23. CDC Healthy Schools, "Whole School, Whole Community, Whole Child (WSCC)," Centers for Disease Control and Prevention, 2018, https://www.cdc.gov/healthyschools/wscc/index.htm. This site includes a graphic representation of the WSCC model.

24. Lewallen TC, Hunt H, Potts-Datema W, et al., "The Whole School, Whole Community, Whole Child Model: A New Approach for Improving Educational Attainment and Healthy Development for Students," *Journal of School Health* 85, no. 11 (2015): 729–39, https://www.ncbi.nlm.nih.gov/pubmed/26440815.

25. Hunt H (guest ed.), "Special Issue: The Whole School, Whole Community, Whole Child Model," *Journal of School Health* 85, no. 11 (November 2015): 729–82, https://onlinelibrary. wiley.com/toc/17461561/85/11.

26. Chriqui J, Stuart-Cassel V, Piekarz-Porter E, et al., "Using State Policy to Create Healthy Schools: Coverage of the Whole School, Whole Community, Whole Child Framework in State Statutes and Regulations, School Year 2017–2018," Child Trends, 2019, https://www. childtrends.org/wp-content/uploads/2019/01/WSCCStatePolicyReportSY2017-18_ ChildTrends_January2019.pdf.

27. Kaiser Permanente, "Thriving Schools," 2019, https://thrivingschools.Kaiser Permanente permanente.org/.

28. Gallup, *State of America's Schools Report* (Washington, DC: Gallup, 2014), www.gallup.com/ file/services/178769/Gallup_Report_--_State_of_Americas_Schools.pdf.

29. Kaiser Permanente, "Resilience in School Environments Project Provides Mental Health and Wellness Support," 2017, https://community.kp.org/stories/story/resilience-in-school-environments-project-provides-mental-health-and-wellness.

30. Washington State University Extension, *CLEAR*, https://extension.wsu.edu/clear/.

31. University of California San Francisco, *UCSF HEARTS: Healthy Environments and Response to Trauma in Schools* (San Francisco: University of California San Francisco, 2019), http:// hearts.ucsf.edu/.

32. Los Angeles Education Partnership, 2018, https://www.laep.org/.

Chapter 5

1. U.S. Department of Labor, Bureau of Labor Statistics, Labor Force Statistics From the Current Population Survey, https://www.bls.gov/cps/cpsaat11b.htm.

2. RWJF's Pioneer Portfolio funds projects that help the Foundation "anticipate the future and consider new and unconventional perspectives and approaches to building a Culture of Health."

3. RWJF describes the initiative as designed to "fund research to better understand the private sector's role in improving economic well-being and community outcomes; build and disseminate evidence to catalyze future private-sector policies and innovations; and spur external efforts to spread and fund these and similar Culture of Health–related innovations."

4. *The Workplace and Health*, National Public Radio, Robert Wood Johnson Foundation, and Harvard T.H. Chan School of Public Health, July 2016, https://www.rwjf.org/en/library/ research/2016/07/the-workplace-and-health.html.

5. Adler D and Tarini P, "How the Future of Work May Impact Our Well-Being," Robert Wood Johnson Foundation, Culture of Health Blog, November 8, 2018, https://www.rwjf.org/en/ blog/2018/09/how-the-future-of-work-may-impact-our-wellbeing.html.

6. *Fortune*, May 21, 2018, http://fortune.com/2018/05/21/fortune-500-companies-2018/.

7. The definition of corporate social performance comes from Wood DJ, "Corporate Social Performance Revisited," *Academy of Management Review* 16, no. 4 (1991): 691–718.

8. Ahn's project "Measuring Corporate Social Performance as Related to Business Organizations' Impact on Public Health and Health Equity" was supported by RWJF Grant ID 74321.

9. Song Z and Baicker K, "Effect of a Workplace Wellness Program on Employee Health and Economic Outcomes: A Randomized Clinical Trial," *JAMA* 32, no. 15 (April 16, 2019): 1491–501, abstract available at https://jamanetwork.com/journals/jama/article-abstract/2730614.

10. The follow-up study, titled "Advancing RWJF's Knowledge of Corporate Disclosure on Social Media of Their Actions Related to Health and/or the Social Determinants of Health," is supported by RWJF Grant ID 75752.

11. More information about the C. Everett Koop National Health Awards is available at http:// thehealthproject.com/award-information-2/.

12. Goetzel's project "Comparing Workers' Health, Medical Expenditures, and Stock Price for Companies That Have and Have Not Invested in Community Health" was supported by RWJF Grant ID 74318.

13. Henke RM, Head MA, Kent KB, et al., "Improvements in an Organization's Culture of Health Reduces Workers' Health Risk Profile and Health Care Utilization," *Journal of Occupational*

and Environmental Medicine 61, no. 2 (February 2019): 96–101, abstract available at https://journals.lww.com/joem/Abstract/2019/02000/Improvements_in_an_Organization_s_Culture_of.2.aspx.

14. Kent KB, Goetzel RZ, Roemer EC, et al., "Developing Two Culture of Health Measurement Tools: Examining Employers' Efforts to Influence Population Health Inside and Outside Company Walls," *Journal of Occupational and Environmental Medicine* 60, no. 12 (December 1, 2018): 1087–97, abstract available at https://journals.lww.com/joem/Citation/2018/12000/Developing_Two_Culture_of_Health_Measurement.6.aspx.

15. Goetzel RZ, Fabius R, Roemer EC, et al., "The Stock Performance of American Companies Investing in a Culture of Health," *American Journal of Health Promotion* 33, no. 3 (March 2019): 439–47, abstract available at https://journals.sagepub.com/doi/abs/10.1177/0890117118824818.

16. "Job Quality and Economic Opportunity in Retail: Key Findings From a National Survey of the Retail Workforce," Center for Popular Democracy, November 2017, https://populardemocracy.org/sites/default/files/DataReport-WebVersion-01-03-18.pdf.

17. U.S. Department of Labor, Bureau of Labor Statistics, Labor Force Characteristics from the Current Population Survey, Table 39, https://www.bls.gov/cps/aa2017/cpsaat39.htm.

18. "Job Quality and Economic Opportunity in Retail."

19. Lambert SJ, Fugiel PJ, and Henly JR, "Precarious Work Schedules Among Early-Career Employees in the U.S.: A National Snapshot," research brief issued by EINet (Employment Instability, Family Well-Being, and Social Policy Network), University of Chicago, 2014, https://ssa.uchicago.edu/sites/default/files/uploads/lambert.fugiel.henly_.precarious_work_schedules.august2014_0.pdf.

20. Williams's project "Analyzing the Impact of Employers' Scheduling Practices on Low-Income Workers' Health and Well-Being" was supported by RWJF Grant ID 74398.

21. Scheiber N, "A Find at Gap: Steady Hours Can Help Workers and Profits," *New York Times*, March 28, 2018.

22. Williams JC, Lambert S, and Kesavan S, "How The Gap Used an App to Give Workers More Control Over Their Schedules." *Harvard Business Review*, December 27, 2017.

23. Williams JC, Kesavan S, and McCorkell L, "Research: When Retail Workers Have Stable Schedules, Sales and Productivity Go Up," *Harvard Business Review*, March 29, 2018.

24. Williams JC, McCorkell L, Lambert S, and Kesavan S, "Who Benefits From Workplace Flexibility? A New Study Tackles Schedule Instability in Retail Jobs," *Slate*, March 28, 2018.

25. Williams JC, Lambert SJ, Kesavan S, et al., "Stable Scheduling Increases Productivity and Sales: The Stable Scheduling Study," March 2018, https://worklifelaw.org/projects/stable-scheduling-study/.

26. *2017 Demographics: Profile of the Military Community*, U.S. Department of Defense, http://download.militaryonesource.mil/12038/MOS/Reports/2017-demographics-report.pdf.

27. Ibid.

28. Qualified Military Available (QMA), Department of Defense, 2017, acquired from the Accession Policy and Joint Advertising, Market Research and Studies teams, U.S. Department of Defense, November 2017.

29. The chairman of the Joint Chiefs of Staff Instruction establishing Total Force Fitness is available at https://www.jcs.mil/Portals/36/Documents/Library/Instructions/3405_01.pdf?ver=2016-02-05-175032-517.

30. For more information about Total Force Domains, see Walter, JAG, "Defining Total Force Fitness for the 21st Century," Samueli Institute, https://apps.dtic.mil/dtic/tr/fulltext/u2/a545537.pdf.

31. Small Business Resilience, UPROSE, https://www.uprose.org/small-business-serv.

Section III

1. López G, Bialik K, and Radford J, "Key Findings About U.S. Immigrants," Pew Research Center, Fact Tank, November 30, 2018, http://www.pewresearch.org/fact-tank/2018/11/30/key-findings-about-u-s-immigrants/.

2. Families USA, https://familiesusa.org/issues/medicaid.

Chapter 6

1. Lee MYH, "Does the United States Really Have 5 Percent of the World's Population and One Quarter of the World's Prisoners?" *Washington Post*, Fact Checker, April 30, 2015, *www.washingtonpost.com/news/fact-checker/wp/2015/04/30/does-the-united-states-really-have-five-percent-of-worlds-population-and-one-quarter-of-the-worlds-prisoners/?noredirect=on&utm_term=.662ebeb01c4b.*

2. "The Sentencing Project: Criminal Justice Facts," The Sentencing Project, Washington, DC, 2017, *www.sentencingproject.org/criminal-justice-facts/.*

3. Gramlich J, "America's Incarceration Rate Is at a Two-Decade Low," Pew Research Center, Fact Tank, May 2, 2018, *www.pewresearch.org/fact-tank/2018/05/02/americas-incarceration-rate-is-at-a-two-decade-low/.*

4. "Sentencing Project: Criminal Justice Facts."

5. Gramlich J, "5 Facts About Crime in the U.S.," Pew Research Center, Fact Tank, January 3, 2019, *www.pewresearch.org/fact-tank/2019/01/03/5-facts-about-crime-in-the-u-s/.*

6. Delaney R, Subramanian R, Shames A, et al., *Reimagining Prison* (New York: Vera Institute of Justice, October 2018), *https://storage.googleapis.com/vera-web-assets/downloads/Publications/reimagining-prison-print-report/legacy_downloads/Reimagining-Prison_FINAL2_digital.pdf.*

7. Acker J, Braveman P, Arkin E, et al., *Mass Incarceration Threatens Health Equity in America* (Princeton, NJ: Robert Wood Johnson Foundation, 2019), *www.rwjf.org/content/dam/farm/reports/issue_briefs/2018/rwjf450812.*

8. *New York City Community Health Profiles Atlas, 2015*, NYC Health, New York, 2015, *www1.nyc.gov/assets/doh/downloads/pdf/data/2015_CHP_Atlas.pdf.*

9. Sampson RJ and Loeffler C, "Punishment's Place: The Local Concentration of Mass Incarceration," *Daedalus* 139, no. 3 (2010): 20–31, *www.ncbi.nlm.nih.gov/pmc/articles/PMC3043762/.*

10. Vera Institute of Justice, Incarceration Trends Project, New York, 2018.

11. Sawyer W, "The Gender Divide: Tracking Women's State Prison Growth," Prison Policy Initiative, January 9, 2018, *www.prisonpolicy.org/reports/women_overtime.html.*

12. Kajstura A, "States of Women's Incarceration: The Global Context 2018," Prison Policy Initiative, June 2018, *www.prisonpolicy.org/global/women/2018.html.*

13. Wakefield S and Wildeman C, "How Parental Incarceration Harms Children and What to Do About It," National Council on Family Relations, *Policy Brief* 3, no. 1 (January 2018), *www.ncfr.org/sites/default/files/2018-01/How%20Parental%20Incarceration%20Harms%20Children%20NCFR%20Policy_Full%20Brief_Jan.%202018_0.pdf.*

14. Wildeman C, Goldman AW, and Turney K, "Parental Incarceration and Child Health in the United States," *Epidemiologic Reviews* 40, no. 1 (2018): 146–56, *https://academic.oup.com/epirev/article-abstract/40/1/146/4964052.*

15. Acker, et al., *Mass Incarceration Threatens Health Equity in America.*

16. Wagner P and Sawyer W, *Mass Incarceration: The Whole Pie 2018* (Northampton, MA: Prison Policy Initiative, 2018), *www.prisonpolicy.org/reports/pie2018.html.*

17. Acker, et al., *Mass Incarceration Threatens Health Equity in America.*

18. "Why Are People in Jail Before Trial?" Pretrial Justice Institute, Rockville, MD, 2018, *www.pretrial.org/get-involved/learn-more/why-we-need-pretrial-reform/.*

19. Wagner and Sawyer, *Mass Incarceration.*

20. McKillup M and Boucher A, "Aging Prison Populations Drive Up Costs," Pew Charitable Trusts, Washington, DC, February 20, 2018, *www.pewtrusts.org/en/research-and-analysis/articles/2018/02/20/aging-prison-populations-drive-up-costs.*

21. Cloud D, *On Life Support: Public Health in the Age of Mass Incarceration* (New York: Vera Institute of Justice, November 2014), *https://storage.googleapis.com/vera-web-assets/downloads/Publications/on-life-support-public-health-in-the-age-of-mass-incarceration/legacy_downloads/on-life-support-public-health-mass-incarceration-report.pdf.*

22. *New York City Community Health Profiles Atlas, 2015.*

23. Nosrati E, Kang-Brown J, Ash M, et al., "Deindustrialization, Incarceration, and Mortality From Diseases of Despair in the United States: County-Level Analysis, 1980–2014," paper presented at Incarceration, a Vera Institute of Justice research symposium, October 2018.

24. *Restoring Promise: A Young Adult Reform Initiative* (New York: Vera Institute of Justice, 2019), *www.vera.org/projects/restoring-promise-young-adult-reform-initiative.*
25. Delaney R, Subramanian R, Shames A, et al., *Reimagining Prison: Executive Summary* (New York: Vera Institute of Justice, October 2018), *https://storage.googleapis.com/vera-web-assets/downloads/Publications/reimagining-prison-print-report/legacy_downloads/Reimagining-Prison_Executive-Summary.pdf.*
26. Whitaker B, "German-Style Program at a Connecticut Maximum Security Prison Emphasizes Rehab for Inmates," *60 Minutes*, CBS News, March 31, 2019, *www.cbsnews.com/news/german-style-true-program-at-cheshire-correctional-institution-emphasizes-rehab-for-inmates-60-minutes/.*
27. *Collateral Costs: Incarceration's Effect on Economic Mobility* (Washington, DC: Pew Charitable Trusts, 2010), *www.pewtrusts.org/~/media/legacy/uploadedfiles/pcs_assets/2010/collateralcosts1pdf.pdf.*
28. *A Shared Sentence: The Devastating Toll of Parental Incarceration on Kids, Families, and Communities* (Baltimore, MD: Annie E. Casey Foundation, 2016), *www.aecf.org/m/resourcedoc/aecf-asharedsentence-2016.pdf#page=7.*
29. Chase-Lansdale PL, Sommer TE, Sabol TJ, et al., "What Are the Effects of a Two-Generation Human Capital Program on Low-Income Parents' Education, Employment, and Psychological Well-Being?," Two-Generation Programs—Policy Brief #1, Ascend at the Aspen Institute, Washington, DC, May 2019, *www.ipr.northwestern.edu/research-areas/child-adolescent/NU2gen/docs/cap-fls-year-1-and-2-findings_brief-i_may-2019.pdf.*
30. Chase-Lansdale PL, Sabol TJ, Sommer TE, et al., "Effects of a Two-Generation Human Capital Program on Low-Income Parents' Education, Employment, and Psychological Well-Being," *Journal of Family Psychology* 33, no. 4 (2019): 433–43, *https://psycnet.apa.org/record/2019-12794-001.*
31. Sommer TE, Schneider W, Sabol TJ, et al., "What Are the Effects of a Two-Generation Human Capital Program on Children's Attendance and Chronic Absence in Head Start?," Two-Generation Programs—Policy Brief #3, Ascend at the Aspen Institute, Washington, DC, May 2019, *www.ipr.northwestern.edu/research-areas/child-adolescent/NU2gen/docs/cap-fls-year-1-and-2-findings_brief-iii_may-2019.pdf.*
32. Sabol TJ, Chor E, Sommer TE, et al. "What Are the Effects of a Two-Generation Human Capital Program on Children's Outcomes in Head Start?," Two-Generation Programs—Policy Brief #2, Ascend at the Aspen Institute, Washington, DC, May 2019, *www.ipr.northwestern.edu/research-areas/child-adolescent/NU2gen/docs/cap-fls-year-1-and-2-findings_brief-ii_may-2019.pdf.*
33. Ibid.
34. *The PATHS® Curriculum*, Channing Bete Company Inc., *www.pathstraining.com/main/curriculum/.*
35. *2017 Point-in-Time Report, Seven-County Metro Denver Region* (Denver: Metro Denver Homeless Initiative, 2017), *https://d3n8a8pro7vhmx.cloudfront.net/mdhi/pages/12/attachments/original/1498599733/2017_Metro_Denver_PIT_Final.pdf?1498599733.*
36. Ibid.
37. Ibid.
38. Covington O, "'Let Us Begin': Ground Broken for Indy Criminal Justice Center," *Indiana Lawyer*, July 12, 2018, *www.theindianalawyer.com/articles/47546-let-us-begin-ground-broken-for-indy-criminal-justice-center.*
39. Runevitch J, "Unique MCAT Program Finds Success on Indy's East Side," WTHR, April 2, 2018, *www.wthr.com/article/unique-mcat-program-finds-success-on-indys-east-side.*

Chapter 6 Spotlight: Fathers Mentoring Fathers

1. See Father Matters, *https://fathermatters.org/.*

Chapter 7

1. "2017 Drug Overdose Deaths," Centers for Disease Control and Prevention, *www.cdc.gov/drugoverdose/data/statedeaths.html.*

2. Hedegaard H, Minino AM, and Warner W, "Drug Overdose Deaths in the United States, 1999–2017," *NCHS Data Brief*, no. 329, November 2018, *www.cdc.gov/nchs/data/databriefs/db329-h.pdf*.

3. Katz J and Sanger-Katz M, "The Numbers Are So Staggering," *New York Times*, November 28, 2018, *www.nytimes.com/interactive/2018/11/29/upshot/fentanyl-drug-overdose-deaths.html*.

4. Plough, AL, *Knowledge to Action: Accelerating Progress in Health, Well-Being, and Equity* (New York: Oxford University Press, 2017), 9–19.

5. Case A and Deaton A, "Rising Morbidity and Mortality in Midlife Among White Non-Hispanic Americans in the 21st Century," *Proceedings of the National Academy of Sciences of the United States of America*, December 8, 2015, *www.pnas.org/content/112/49/15078*.

6. "Key Substance Use and Mental Health Indicators in the United States: Results from the 2017 National Survey on Drug Use and Health," Substance Abuse and Mental Health Services Administration, U.S. Department of Health and Human Services, *www.samhsa.gov/data/report/2017-nsduh-annual-national-report*.

7. Hedegaard, Minino, and Warner, "Drug Overdose Deaths in the United States."

8. "U.S. Opioid Prescribing Rate Maps," Center for Disease Control and Prevention, *www.cdc.gov/drugoverdose/maps/rxrate-maps.html*.

9. "U.S. Opioid Deaths Jump Fourfold in 20 Years; Epidemic Shifts to Eastern States," Stanford University Medicine, February 22, 2019, *https://med.stanford.edu/news/all-news/2019/02/u-s-opioid-deaths-jump-fourfold-in-20-years.html*.

10. "Life in Rural America," National Public Radio, the Robert Wood Johnson Foundation, the Harvard T.H. Chan School of Public Health, October 1, 2018, *www.rwjf.org/content/dam/farm/reports/surveys_and_polls/2018/rwjf449263*.

11. Ibid.

12. "Rural Communities in Crisis," Bloomberg American Health Initiative, *https://americanhealth.jhu.edu/article/rural-communities-crisis*.

13. Graham C, "Well-Being: From Measures to Action," *Sharing Knowledge to Build a Culture of Health* conference, Robert Wood Johnson Foundation, 2018, plenary session.

14. "Communities in Crisis: Local Responses to Behavioral Health Challenges," Manatt Health with funding from Robert Wood Johnson Foundation, *www.rwjf.org/en/library/research/2017/10/communities-in-crisis--local-responses-to-behavioral-health-challenges.html*.

15. "Opioid Addiction Treatment Behind Bars," ScienceDaily, February 14, 2018, *www.sciencedaily.com/releases/2018/02/180214111109.htm*.

16. "Increased Narcan Availability Evokes Ethical Debate," Healio, Primary Care, *www.healio.com/family-medicine/addiction/news/online/%7Bcc6f0744-e492-4997-97ca-2443e2d2597c%7D/increased-narcan-availability-evokes-ethical-debate*.

17. Katz J, "Why a City at the Center of the Opioid Crisis Gave Up a Tool to Fight It," *New York Times*, April 27, 2018, *www.nytimes.com/interactive/2018/04/27/upshot/charleston-opioid-crisis-needle-exchange.html*.

18. "Provisional Drug Overdose Death Counts," National Center for Health Statistics, Centers for Disease Control and Prevention, *www.cdc.gov/nchs/nvss/vsrr/drug-overdose-data.htm*.

19. "Opioid Addiction Treatment Behind Bars Reduced Post-Incarceration Overdose Deaths in Rhode Island," ScienceDaily, February 14, 2018, *www.sciencedaily.com/releases/2018/02/180214111109.htm*.

20. "A Blueprint for Transforming Opioid Use Disorder Treatment in Delaware," Johns Hopkins Bloomberg School of Public Health and the Bloomberg American Health Initiative, July 2018, *https://dhss.delaware.gov/dhss/files/johnshopkinsrep.pdf*.

21. "What States Need to Know About PDMPs," Centers for Disease Control and Prevention, *www.cdc.gov/drugoverdose/pdmp/states.html*.

22. Goodnough A, Katz J, and Sanger-Katz M, "Drug Overdose Deaths Drop in U.S. for First Time Since 1990," *New York Times*, July 17, 2019, *www.nytimes.com/interactive/2019/07/17/upshot/drug-overdose-deaths-fall.html*.

23. *www.pewtrusts.org/-/media/assets/2019/07/core_rli_071219.pdf?la=en&hash=75B0504658 68E2BED74A8D9316A0BD14CA7CAD95*

Chapter 8

1. Zong J, Batalova J, and Hallock J, "Frequently Requested Statistics on Immigrants and Immigration in the United States," Migration Information Source Spotlight, February 8, 2018, *www.migrationpolicy.org/article/frequently-requested-statistics-immigrants-and-immigration-united-states*.
2. López G, Bialik K, and Radford J, "Key Findings About U.S. Immigrants," Pew Research Center, Fact Tank, November 30, 2018, *www.pewresearch.org/fact-tank/2018/11/30/key-findings-about-u-s-immigrants/*.
3. "Children of Immigrants Data Tool," Urban Institute, Washington, DC, 2019, *http://datatool.urban.org/charts/datatool/pages.cfm*.
4. López, Bialik, and Radford, "Key Findings About U.S. Immigrants."
5. Passel JS and Cohn D, "U.S. Unauthorized Immigrant Total Dips to Lowest Level in a Decade," Pew Research Center, *Hispanic Trends*, November 27, 2018, *www.pewhispanic.org/2018/11/27/u-s-unauthorized-immigrant-total-dips-to-lowest-level-in-a-decade/*.
6. "Table 11. Persons Obtaining Lawful Permanent Resident Status by Broad Class of Admission and Region and Country of Last Residence: Fiscal Year 2017," *2017 Yearbook of Immigration Status*, Department of Homeland Security, 2018, *www.dhs.gov/immigration-statistics/yearbook/2017/table11*.
7. López, Bialik, and Radford, "Key Findings About U.S. Immigrants."
8. Ramakrishnan K and Shah S, "One Out of Every 7 Asian Immigrants Is Undocumented," Data Bits: A Blog for AAPI Data, September 8, 2017, *http://aapidata.com/blog/asian-undoc-1in7/*.
9. López, Bialik, and Radford, "Key Findings About U.S. Immigrants."
10. "Health Status and Access to Care," in *The Integration of Immigrants into American Society* (Washington, DC: National Academies of Sciences, Engineering, and Medicine, 2015), *www.nap.edu/read/21746/chapter/11*.
11. Zallman L, Woolhandler S, Himmelstein D, et al., "Immigrants Contributed an Estimated $115.2 Billion More to the Medicare Trust Fund Than They Took Out in 2002–09," *Health Affairs* 32, no. 6 (2013), *www.healthaffairs.org/doi/full/10.1377/hlthaff.2012.1223*.
12. Brooks T, Wagnerman K, Argtiga S, et al., "Medicaid and CHIP Eligibility, Enrollment, Renewal, and Cost Sharing Policies as of January 2018: Findings From a 50-State Survey," Henry J. Kaiser Family Foundation, 2018, *www.kff.org/medicaid/report/medicaid-and-chip-eligibility-enrollment-renewal-and-cost-sharing-policies-as-of-january-2018-findings-from-a-50-state-survey/*.
13. "Status of State Medicaid Expansion Decisions: Interactive Map," Henry J. Kaiser Family Foundation, April 9, 2019, *www.kff.org/medicaid/issue-brief/status-of-state-medicaid-expansion-decisions-interactive-map/*.
14. Bhatt CB and Beck-Sagué CM, "Medicaid Expansion and Infant Mortality in the United States," *American Journal of Public Health* 108, no. 4 (2018): 565–67, *www.ncbi.nlm.nih.gov/pmc/articles/PMC5844390/*.
15. Brooks, Wagnerman, Argtiga, and Cornachione, "Medicaid and CHIP Eligibility."
16. Gutierrez M, "Gov. Gavin Newsom Proposes Healthcare Mandate, Medi-Cal Expansion to More Immigrants Without Legal Status," *Los Angeles Times*, January 7, 2019, *www.latimes.com/politics/la-pol-ca-gavin-newsom-healthcare-proposal-20190107-story.html*.
17. Associated Press, "Mayor Says NYC Will Expand Health Coverage to 600,000 People," *New York Times*, January 8, 2019, *www.nytimes.com/aponline/2019/01/08/nyregion/ap-us-nyc-public-health-care.html*.
18. Information in this section is from the Immigrant Legal Resource Center, *www.ilrc.org/public-charge*.
19. "Inadmissibility on Public Charge Grounds." Federal Register: August 14, 2019, printed page 41304.
20. Ibid, printed page 41305.
21. Shear MD and Sullivan E. "Trump Policy Favors Wealthier Immigrants for Green Cards." *New York Times*: August 12, 2019.

22. Flores G, "Families Facing Language Barriers in Healthcare: When Will Policy Catch Up With the Demographics and Evidence?" *Journal of Pediatrics* 164, no. 6 (June 2014): 1261–64, *www.jpeds.com/article/S0022-3476(14)00173-5/fulltext*.

23. Batalova J and Zong J, "Language Diversity and English Proficiency in the United States," Migration Information Source Spotlight, November 11, 2016, *www.migrationpolicy.org/article/language-diversity-and-english-proficiency-united-states*.

24. Jimenez M, Martinez Alcarez E, Williams J, et al., "Access to Developmental Pediatrics Evaluations for At-Risk Children," *Journal of Developmental & Behavioral Pediatrics* 38, no. 3 (2017): 228–32, *https://journals.lww.com/jrnldbp/Citation/2017/04000/Access_to_Developmental_Pediatrics_Evaluations_for.8.aspx*.

25. Lion KC, Thompson DA, Cowden JD, et al., "Clinical Spanish Use and Language Proficiency Testing Among Pediatric Residents," *Academic Medicine* 88, no. 10 (2013): 1478–84, *www.ncbi.nlm.nih.gov/pubmed/23969350*.

26. Ohtani A, Suzuki T, Takeuchi H, et al., "Language Barriers and Access to Psychiatric Care: A Systematic Review," *Psychiatric Services* 66, no. 8 (2015): 798–805, *www.ncbi.nlm.nih.gov/pubmed/25930043*.

27. "Access to Adolescent Mental Health Care," Office of Adolescent Health, U.S. Department of Health and Human Services, 2018, *www.hhs.gov/ash/oah/adolescent-development/mental-health/access-adolescent-mental-health-care/index.html*.

28. Harper B and O'Boyle B, "Explainer: What Is DACA?," Americas Society / Council of the Americas, New York, September 13, 2018, *www.as-coa.org/articles/explainer-what-daca?gclid=EAIaIQobChMIo9-0ypnw3wIVl4zICh0-yw3vEAAYAyAAEgLG_fD_BwE*.

29. Lopez G and Krogstad JM, "Key Facts About Unauthorized Immigrants Enrolled in DACA," Pew Research Center, Fact Tank, September 25, 2017, *www.pewresearch.org/fact-tank/2017/09/25/key-facts-about-unauthorized-immigrants-enrolled-in-daca/*.

30. Hainmueller J, Lawrence D, Martén L, et al., "Protecting Unauthorized Immigrant Mothers Improves Their Children's Mental Health," *Science* 357, no. 6355 (2017): 1041–44, *https://europepmc.org/backend/ptpmcrender.fcgi?accid=PMC5990252&blobtype=pdf*.

31. Swartz JJ, Hainmueller J, Lawrence D, et al., "Expanding Prenatal Care to Unauthorized Immigrant Women and the Effects on Infant Health," *Obstetrics & Gynecology* 130, no. 5 (2017): 938–45, *https://journals.lww.com/greenjournal/fulltext/2017/11000/Expanding_Prenatal_Care_to_Unauthorized_Immigrant.2.aspx*.

32. Swartz JJ, Hainmueller J, Lawrence D, et al., "Oregon's Expansion of Prenatal Care Improved Utilization Among Immigrant Women," *Maternal and Child Health Journal* 23, no. 2 (2019): 173–82, *www.ncbi.nlm.nih.gov/pubmed/30039326*.

Chapter 9

1. "Helping Communities Prepare For, Withstand, and Recover From Disaster," Robert Wood Johnson Foundation, Culture of Health Blog, March 7, 2018. *www.rwjf.org/en/blog/2018/03/help-communities-prepare-for-and-recover-from-disaster.html*.

2. Plough AL, "The Impact of Climate Change on Health and Equity," Robert Wood Johnson Foundation, Culture of Health Blog, June 22, 2016, *www.rwjf.org/en/blog/2016/06/what_does_climatech.html*.

3. UN International Panel on Climate Change, "Global Warming of 1.5 °C," *www.ipcc.ch/sr15/*.

4. Mooney C and Dennis B, "The World Has Just Over a Decade to Get Climate Change Under Control, UN Scientists Say," *Washington Post*, October 7, 2018, *www.washingtonpost.com/energy-environment/2018/10/08/world-has-only-years-get-climate-change-under-control-un-scientists-say/?utm_term=.be97508894c1*.

5. Ibid.

6. Ibid.

7. Editorial Board, "The Green New Deal Is Better Than Our Climate Nightmare," *New York Times*, February 23, 2019, *www.nytimes.com/2019/02/23/opinion/green-new-deal-climate-democrats.html*.

8. Reidmiller DR, Avery CW, Easterling DR, et al., *Impacts, Risks, and Adaptation in the United States: Fourth National Climate Assessment, Volume II: Report-in-Brief*, U.S. Global Change Research Program, Washington, DC, *https://nca2018.globalchange.gov/downloads/NCA4_ Report-in-Brief.pdf*.
9. Sengupta S and Pierre-Louis K, "Study Warns of Cascading Health Risks From the Changing Climate," *New York Times*, November 28, 2018, *www.nytimes.com/2018/11/28/climate/ climate-change-health.html*.
10. Ibid.
11. Dennis B and Mooney C, "Major Trump Administration Climate Report Says Damages Are 'Intensifying Across the Country,'" *Washington Post*, November 23, 2018, *www.washingtonpost. com/energy-environment/2018/11/23/major-trump-administration-climate-report-says-damages-are-intensifying-across-country/?utm_term=.cb0663e89835*.
12. Ibid.
13. "Health and Climate Change Landscape Assessment," Climate Central, with funding from Robert Wood Johnson Foundation, August 18, 2017, *www.rwjf.org/en/library/research/ 2017/08/health-and-climate-change-landscape-assessment.html*.
14. Ibid.
15. For number of deaths, see George Washington University Milken Institute School of Public Health, independent report, August 28, 2018, *https://publichealth.gwu.edu/content/gw-report-delivers-recommendations-aimed-preparing-puerto-rico-hurricane-season*. For damage, see Puerto Rican government report to Congress, August 9, 2018, *www.npr.org/2018/08/09/ 637230089/puerto-rico-estimates-it-will-cost-139-billion-to-fully-recover-from-hurricane-maria*.
16. Climate Justice Center, post–Superstorm Sandy in Sunset Park, *www.uprose.org/climate-justice*.
17. Gill DA, Ritchie LA, and Picou JS, "Litigation and Settlements Following the Exxon Valdez and BP Deepwater Horizon Oil Spills: When the Disasters Are Crimes," in *Crime and Criminal Justice in Disasters* (Durham, NC: Carolina Academic Press, 2015).
18. Ritchie LA, Gill DA, and Long MA, "Mitigating Litigating: An Examination of Psychosocial Impacts of Compensation Processes Associated With the 2010 BP Deepwater Horizon Oil Spill," *Risk Analysis* 38 (November 8, 2018).
19. Ritchie LA, Little J, Campbell NM, "Resources Loss and Psychosocial Stress in the Aftermath of the 2008 Tennessee Valley Authority Coal Ash Spill," *International Journal of Mass Emergencies and Disasters* 36, no. 2 (August 2018): 179–207.
20. Ritchie LA, Gill DA, Picoa JS, "The BP Disaster as an *Exxon Valdez* Rerun," *Contexts* 10, no. 3 (Summer 2011): 30–35, *https://journals.sagepub.com/doi/full/10.1177/1536504211418454*.
21. Gill, Ritchie, and Picou, "Litigation and Settlements Following the Exxon Valdez and BP Deepwater Horizon Oil Spills."
22. Ritchie, Gill, and Long, "Mitigating Litigating."
23. Ibid.
24. Gill, Ritchie, and Picou, "Litigation and Settlements Following the Exxon Valdez and BP Deepwater Horizon Oil Spills."
25. Ibid.
26. The Gulf Research Program, *www.nationalacademies.org/gulf/about/index.html*.
27. Thriving Communities Grant Awards, the Gulf Research Project, National Academics of Sciences, Engineering, and Medicine, *www.nas.edu/gulf/grants/awards/thriving-communities/ index.htm#thriving1*.
28. "National Academics' Gulf Research Program and RWJF Award $10.8 Million to Build Healthy, Resilient Coastal Communities," July 18, 2017, www.rwjf.org/en/library/articles-and-news/2017/07/national-academies-gulf-research-program-and-rwjf-award-10-8-million-to-build-healthy-resilient-coastal-communities.html.
29. Costigan T, "What's the Formula for Community Resilience?" Robert Wood Johnson Foundation, Culture of Health Blog, August 1, 2016, *www.rwjf.org/en/blog/2016/07/what_ s_the_formulaf.html*.
30. "National Academics' Gulf Research Program and RWJF Award $10.8 Million to Build Healthy, Resilient Coastal Communities."
31. Small Business Resilience, UPROSE, *www.uprose.org/small-business-serv*.
32. "Help Communities Prepare For, Withstand, and Recover From Disaster."

33. "Health and Climate Solutions 2018 Call for Proposals," Robert Wood Johnson Foundation, December 17, 2018, *www.rwjf.org/en/library/funding-opportunities/2018/health-and-climate-solutions-hub.html.*

34. Plough, "Impact of Climate Change on Health and Equity."

Chapter 9 Spotlight: A Just Recovery for Puerto Rico

1. "Our Power Puerto Rico Campaign," Climate Justice Alliance, *https://climatejusticealliance.org/our-power-puerto-rico/.*

2. Yeampierre E and Klein N, "Imagine a Puerto Rican Recovery Designed by Puerto Ricans," *The Intercept,* October 20, 2017, *https://theintercept.com/2017/10/20/puerto-rico-hurricane-debt-relief/.*

3. "OurPowerPR Solidarity Brigades Rebuild Puerto Rico," Climate Justice Alliance, January 25, 2018, *https://climatejusticealliance.org/ourpowerpr-solidarity-brigades-rebuild-puerto-rico/.*

4. "Support Our Power," Climate Justice Alliance, *https://climatejusticealliance.org/our-power-puerto-rico/.*

5. "#OurPower PRNYC Marks One-Year Mark of Hurricane Maria: 1000+ Leaders, Artists, Activists Unite to Demand Just Recovery for Puerto Rico," Climate Justice Alliance press release, September 20, 2018, *https://climatejusticealliance.org/ourpowerprnyc-marks-one-year-mark-hurricane-maria-1000-leaders-artists-activists-unite-demand-justrecovery-puerto-rico/.*

Chapter 10

1. "Health Care Without Harm's Research Collaborative," Robert Wood Johnson Foundation Program Results Report, March 25, 2013, *www.rwjf.org/en/library/research/2012/01/health-care-without-harm-s-research-collaborative.html.*

2. Gerwig K, *Greening Health Care: How Hospitals Can Heal the Planet* (New York: Oxford University Press, 2015), 5–7.

3. "Health and Climate Change Landscape Assessment."

4. Ibid.

5. Eckelman MJ and Sherman S, "Environmental Impacts of the U.S. Health Care System and Effects on Public Health," *PLOS ONE* 11, no. 6 (2016): 4, *https://journals.plos.org/plosone/article?id=10.1371/journal.pone.0157014.*

6. Gerwig, *Greening Health Care,* 5.

7. Ibid., 6.

8. Gary Cohen, interview with Judith Nemes, 2011, quoted in ibid., 7.

9. "Our Story," Practice Greenhealth, *https://practicegreenhealth.org/about/history.*

10. Gerwig, *Greening Health Care,* 7.

11. "Health Care Without Harm's Research Collaborative."

12. Highlights and descriptive copy adopted (in some cases verbatim) from "History and Victories, Success Stories," Health Care Without Harm, *https://noharm-uscanada.org/content/us-canada/history-and-victories.*

13. "Restorative Health Care: A Resilient and Restorative Health Care Sector," Health Care Without Harm, *https://noharm-uscanada.org/issues/us-canada/restorative-health-care.*

14. "Kaiser Permanente Finalizes Agreement to Enable Carbon Neutrality in 2020," Kaiser Permanente press release, September 10, 2018, *https://share.kaiserpermanente.org/article/kaiser-permanente-finalizes-agreement-to-enable-carbon-neutrality-in-2020/.*

15. "An Appetite for Sustainable Food: Making the Climate Connection," Kaiser Permanente, October 31, 2018, *https://share.kaiserpermanente.org/article/an-appetite-for-sustainable-food-making-the-climate-connection/.*

16. "What We Do," Healthier Hospitals Initiative, January 25, 2012, *www.healthierhospitals.org/about-hh/what-we-do.*

17. "Health and Climate Change Landscape Assessment."

18. Health care commitments at the Global Climate Action Summit, September 2018, *https://noharm-uscanada.org/documents/health-care-commitments-global-climate-action-summit.*

19. "Moving to Renewable Energy Is the Biggest Health Intervention We Can Make," Health Care Without Harm, November 9, 2018, *https://noharm-uscanada.org/articles/news/us-canada/'moving-renewable-energy-biggest-health-intervention-we-can-make.*

20. "68 of the Greenest Hospitals in America, 2018," Becker's Healthcare, *www.beckershospitalreview.com/lists/68-of-the-greenest-hospitals-in-america-2018.html.*

21. "Health Care Without Harm's Research Collaborative."

22. Job posting for Program Officer (REL), Transforming Health and Health Care Systems, The Robert Wood Johnson Foundation, *www.rwjf.org/en/about-rwjf/job-opportunities/program-officer-rel-thhcs.html.*

23. "Comments From Richard Besser on the Surgeon General's Call to Action, 'Community Health and Prosperity,'" Robert Wood Johnson Foundation, November 5, 2018, *www.rwjf.org/en/library/articles-and-news/2018/10/comments-from-richard-besser-on-the-surgeon-generals-call-to-action-community-health-and-prosperity.html.*

Chapter 11

1. "Status of State Medicaid Expansion Decisions," Kaiser Family Foundation, *www.kff.org/medicaid/issue-brief/status-of-state-medicaid-expansion-decisions-interactive-map/.*

2. "April 2019 Medicaid & CHIP Enrollment Data Highlights," Medicaid.gov, *www.medicaid.gov/medicaid/program-information/medicaid-and-chip-enrollment-data/report-highlights/index.html.*

3. "Medicaid," Families USA, *https://familiesusa.org/issues/medicaid.*

4. "Total Medicaid Spending," Kaiser Family Foundation, *www.kff.org/medicaid/state-indicator/total-medicaid-spending/?currentTimeframe=0&sortModel=%7B%22colId%22:%22Location%22,%22sort%22:%22asc%22%7Dspending/?currentTimeframe=0&sortModel=%7B%22colId%22:%22Location%22,%22sort%22:%22asc%22%7D.*

5. "Federal Medical Assistance Percentage for Medicaid," Kaiser Family Foundation, *www.kff.org/medicaid/state-indicator/federal-matching-rate-and-multiplier/?currentTimeframe=0&sortModel=%7B%22colId%22:%22Location%22,%22sort%22:%22asc%22%7D.*

6. Paradise J and Ross DC, "Linking Medicaid and Supportive Housing: Opportunities and On-the-Ground Examples," Kaiser Family Foundation, January 27, 2017, *http://files.kff.org/attachment/Issue-Brief-Linking-Medicaid-and-Supportive-Housing-Opportunities-and-On-the-Ground-Examples.*

7. "Coverage of Housing-Related Activities and Services for Individuals with Disabilities," Center for Medicare and Medicaid Services, *www.medicaid.gov/federal-policy-guidance/downloads/cib-06-26-2015.pdf.*

8. "Total Medicare MCOs, 2017," Kaiser Family Foundation, *www.kff.org/medicaid/state-indicator/total-medicaid-mcos/?activeTab=map&currentTimeframe=0&selectedDistributions=total-medicaid-mcos&sortModel=%7B%22colId%22:%22Location%22,%22sort%22:%22asc%22%7D.*

9. "Medicaid Waiver Tracker: Approved and Pending Waivers by State," Kaiser Family Foundation, June 13, 2019, *www.kff.org/medicaid/issue-brief/medicaid-waiver-tracker-approved-and-pending-section-1115-waivers-by-state/.*

10. "New Service Delivery Opportunities for Individuals With a Substance Use Disorder," Centers for Medicare & Medicaid Services, July 27, 2015, *www.medicaid.gov/federal-policy-guidance/downloads/SMD15003.pdf.*

11. "West Virginia's New Medicaid Waiver Promotes Medicaid Objectives," Center on Budget and Policy Priorities, October 24, 2017, *www.cbpp.org/blog/west-virginias-new-medicaid-waiver-promotes-medicaid-objectives.*

12. West Virginia Bureau for Medical Services, "Substance Use Disorder (SUD) Waiver," *https://dhhr.wv.gov/bms/Programs/WaiverPrograms/Pages/Substance-Use-Disorder-(SUD)-Waiver-.aspx.*

13. RWJF Opioid Challenge, *www.opioidchallenge.com*; Muoio D, "Robert Wood Johnson Foundation Names Winners of $50,000 AI, Opioid Challenges," *Mobi Health News,* September 19, 2018, *www.mobihealthnews.com/content/robert-wood-johnson-foundation-names-winners-50000-ai-opioid-challenges.*

Chapter 11 Spotlight: A Private Insurer Tackles Social Determinants

1. Masterson L, "UnitedHealth Sees Membership, Revenue up in Q1," Healthcare Dive, April 17, 2018, *www.healthcaredive.com/news/unitedhealth-optum-q1-2018/521523/*.
2. Fuentevilla was chief medical officer of UnitedHealthcare's Community and State Division until April 2018. She is currently chief medical officer, Optum Population Health Solutions, a companion company to UnitedHealthcare. Both companies fall under the umbrella of UnitedHealth Group.

INDEX

Page numbers followed by *f* indicate figures.
For the benefit of digital users, indexed terms that span two pages (e.g., 52–53) may, on occasion, appear on only one of those pages.